Breast *Easy*

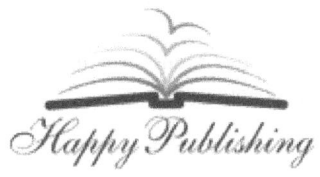

Copyright © 2017 by Happy Publishing and Erica Glessing

First Edition

ISBN: 978-0-9961712-4-3

Cover design by Melinda Asztalos
http://www.wholisticdesigner.com/

Interior design by Noel Morado

No part of this publication may be translated, reproduced or transmitted in any form without prior permission in writing from the publisher.

All of the contributors in this publication have granted permission for inclusion.

Product trade names or trademarks mentioned throughout this publication remain property of their respective owners.

Published by Happy Publishing, HappyPublishing.net

INTRODUCTION

Dear Reader,

The questions that generated and created this book stemmed from a question I asked myself one morning. "How can I expand beyond what I thought was possible?" And the title floated into my consciousness, in that space between sleep and waking. "Breast Easy."

What? No! I can't write about breasts!

No! I am not at ease with my breasts!

That's the one part of my body I have always tried to hide.

That's the one part of my body I have always been ashamed about. Well, I shouldn't say always. There was a brief month or two at age 13 when they first appeared that I thought they were pretty cool. Then the jealousy of the girls and the lecherous eyes of the men and the judgment of others stepped in and I became miserable, knowing my body had the potency to change others in front of my eyes.

So this book had one intention – to create a space for consciousness and the experience of bodies in an all new way. The stories are beyond my expectations and I am indeed honored to present to you – stories about breasts! Lots of sizes, shapes, colors and connectivities. May it warm your heart and turn you on, turn you up, make you laugh, and make you cry, and awaken some awareness inside of you that perhaps was dormant or perhaps you were waiting to find that you indeed, are not alone. You might even find "your tribe."

Thank you to the brave authors willing to be in a 'boobie book' as we joked about it behind the scenes! To your beautiful beingness, women and men alike, and to breasts of every and each possible shape, size, form and consciousness!

Erica Glessing
CEO, Happy Publishing

TABLE OF CONTENTS

Introduction 3

CHAPTER 1   Dear Breasts 7
    Jennifer Nicole Marco

CHAPTER 2   The Heart Path from the Sexy Implants 13
    Cameo Haag

CHAPTER 3   Well, I Never… 25
    Leslie Lang

CHAPTER 4   Breasts: The Key to Feminine Vitality 33
    Dr. Kim D'Eramo

CHAPTER 5   Having Rich Breasts is an Honor 45
    Nicole Richardson

CHAPTER 6   Bye Bye Bra, Hello Freedom! 53
    Elisabeth Schweiger

CHAPTER 7   TURN IT UP! TURN IT UP! 61
  Kim Coleman

CHAPTER 8   A Model Wears Her Breasts Wild 73
  Jennilynne Coley

CHAPTER 9   Vageni 83
  Jeni Griffith Burgess

CHAPTER 10   I Love My Breasts! 93
  Jennifer Lamkins

CHAPTER 11   Having It All 103
  Brittany Rogozinski

CHAPTER 12   Bosom Buddies: Becoming BFFs
  with your Breasts 109
  Julie Oreson Perkins

CHAPTER 13   The Key to Loving the Goddess You Be 123
  Tanya Desaulniers

CHAPTER 14   It's Not Easy Being Gee-zy 133
  Erica Glessing

CHAPTER 1
DEAR BREASTS

Jennifer Nicole Marco

Dear Breasts,

*W*e have had quite the journey through being on a flat-chested girl who was the youngest student in her class, to the somewhat embarrassed college freshman, to the 20 something singer who traveled around the country singing her heart out, to the married woman experiencing her first real sexual relationship.

Then we created a whole new experience, which is motherhood. Oh, how mother changed us from being somewhat manageable to being the ever-increasing supply of life, warmth, nourishment, comfort and milk! Lactation is not for the faint of heart! Possessing mammary glands and then actively using them for 70 straight months is a powerful testament to what breasts CAN do.

From waking up in the morning with an overflow of liquid to falling asleep at night with my resting child, breastfeeding changed me from the outside in and the inside out. I accepted this new part of myself, growing and decreasing daily, this 24-hour process of expansion and

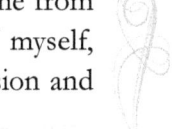

contraction, and it was all to sustain the lives on the wonderful, exquisite creations known as my children.

Though birth in and of itself was a miracle, breastfeeding was the gift that kept giving and giving, through years of midnight feedings, comfort snuggling, toothache soothing and love all contained in the body a girl who is now a woman, the mama bear who gave up fashion for function, who changed her life as a public speaker, singer and coach, all for the sake of providing something precious for her precious ones.

Breastfeeding in the 2000s wasn't exactly the height of couture, designer wear for women who wanted to look trendy and stylish. I traded in my dry clean-only suits and business outfits for wash and wear clothing that sometimes didn't make it to the washing machine.

Pumping proved to be another witness of the capacity of what breasts can really do. The very first night I was home from the hospital with my newborn daughter, she was crying that mournful, starved cry, and I desperately attempted to assemble a cheap, plastic, 15-dollar pump in the middle of the night. My baby wouldn't latch, and I didn't want to feed her formula that evening, so I did my best to find a solution.

Though the pump was not a medical grade, dual action milk machine, it worked well enough to get the flow of milk to begin, and then I tried one last time to team up with my daughter and help her latch on to me. I felt a new and bizarre sense of awe as I lifted her tiny body to my breast and she suddenly and successfully began drinking. In that moment, I released my first post-partum ugly cry of tears, and began a boob bond for nearly two years.

During that time, I also pumped milk for her and for the baby who was joining the family. I had another pregnancy that ended at around 14 weeks gestation and continued to pump for my daughter and the baby whose arrival we eagerly anticipated. The gift of my milk was becoming even more obvious and necessary in ways that I hadn't considered. I had taken for granted the fact that I could actually produce milk easily when other women struggled. After pumping for both babies, I learned that I was pregnant again, and my second daughter arrived in her adorable glory.

She and I had the longest nursing relationship, and I loved every minute of the time with her, though I did feel overwhelmed and exhausted. After the births of both of my daughters, my body quickly released weight and I was in my pre-pregnancy clothes within weeks. I was still nursing my second daughter when I became pregnant with my third child, who is a boy.

My body really struggled during that pregnancy, and I fought a long and difficult fight to bring my baby boy into the world. My ability to move much or exercise was very limited, and I gained 100 pounds. My breasts grew from a 34 B bra size to a 38 or 40 D, depending on the bra, and then I became even larger after giving birth.

I had never been so full-busted or felt like such a prisoner in my own body. The weight didn't come off quickly. After my son was a year old, I still weighed 220 pounds and hardly recognized myself in a mirror. Our breastfeeding experience was very different than what I experienced with my daughters, because my son couldn't tolerate dairy or acidic foods.

After a visit to a naturopathic doctor, I changed my diet drastically, and my baby began to adapt to the changes, and he started to gain weight and thrive. For nine months, I only ate chicken and vegetables, which was an additional sacrifice, because I love food and had a large extended family through marriage that loved food, too. I really love chocolate and sweet things, but I was willing to do anything to help my son. I just intuitively knew that he needed breast milk, so I worked hard to produce it.

After our breastfeeding relationship ended, I started releasing weight, too. I went from 240 pounds at the end of my pregnancy to 140 pounds, and from a size 18/20 to a size 4. And of course, my breasts were the first obvious body part to shift and morph.

About six months after reaching my lightest weight, I chose to become a single mother, and then I was faced another interesting choice. Do I get implants or not? After breastfeeding three children, pumping for another baby, and ending a marriage and living on my own, I wondered what to do next with my life, which lead me to a very inquisitive question. I asked myself, "What if I never had to be pretty again?"

Though I understand that many choose implants for themselves, in my mind and spirit, I could not differentiate between myself and the need to have large breasts for the sake of being attractive and desirable to someone else.

So, instead of choosing the aesthetic route, I chose to look inward, towards self discovery, and to ask questions such as "Whose ideas IS this?" "Who told me that my breasts need to be a certain size?" Who told me that I have to be any certain way to be legitimate as a woman?

What would happen if I never had to be pretty again? Because in my world, pretty equals desirable, which equals lovable, and I was seeking love from something outside of myself to validate something inside of me.

So, I dated and had several serious relationships and ended them all, because I could never wrap my head around the merging of two spaces into one space, or two lives into one life. Once I detached from romance, the attachment to beauty for another's sake decreased, and I found yet another new space to live in that no longer required male validation, acceptance or desirability, because I was desirable to myself, in my own body and being.

I started to celebrate what my body has done. I have sustained the lives of four human beings by producing a nutritious substance, and through touch, time, energy, effort and sacrifice. I've sung in front of stadiums, arenas and amazing concert halls. I've contributed to the world through coaching, retreats, Access Bars, writing and through friendship and connection.

And through it all, I've found the love inside myself that I was always in search of. I never needed to be a certain cup size. I just needed to be ME... beautiful, complete me!

Jennifer Nicole Marco

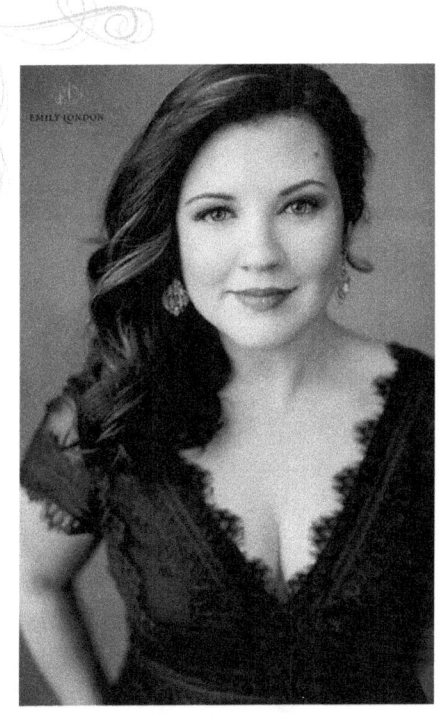

Jennifer Marco *is a professional singer, speaker, coach and Access Consciousness® Bars facilitator. She has been a featured vocalist on 350 studio projects, and loves to inspire and empower women. You can find her on Facebook – Jennifer Nicole Marco.*

CHAPTER 2
THE HEART PATH FROM SEXY IMPLANTS

Cameo Haag

I woke up with great anticipation this morning. The day was finally here. I have been planning, prepping, preparing and pondering what this day would look like for years. I felt excited and scared. I felt happy and sad. I felt confident as well as insecure. I had thoughts racing around my head. What would they look like? How would they feel? Would I like them? Would my husband like them? What size are they going to be? This day was September 8th, 2016 and it was the day I was scheduled to get my breast implants removed. Yes I said removed.

On this day I had my 475 CC saline implants, over the muscle, explanted from my body! For 10.5 years I have been carrying these saline bags with me everywhere I went but today I was free. I was free from the feeling that I was not 100 percent authentically me. I was free from the feeling of pins and needles down my arms. I was free from the constant feeling of always being tired. I was free from the weight on my chest that didn't allow me to take a full, deep breath but most of all I was free from the constant feeling that something wasn't allowing me to fully give or receive love. I am free!

I wanted to share this journey as I have come to realize that a big part of the reason I had my breasts implants put in was to protect my heart. Of course I also wanted to look super-hot with big, nice, fully rounded beautiful boobs and I did. I looked great in that little black dress and I also turned heads in jeans and a T-shirt but as I am healing I know that I chose to get breast implants to guard my heart. They are the perfect protector. They were like the security guards that stands at the entrance of the club deciding who gets in and who must wait in line. The interesting thing about these security guards were they wouldn't allow me to leave either.

I use this analogy as I have always felt trapped, stuck and unable to expand inside my own greatness. Almost as if anytime I expanded I would hit up against something hard and solid, something that would not allow me to express my love to the fullest or receive others love to the fullest. This something was my breast implants.

I absolutely believe that we are spiritual beings having a human experience. So this experience has been life transforming for me. It has shifted my beliefs and awakened me to the powerful woman I am with or without super hooters.

I started asking myself questions. Questions such as...

Why did I want implants? What did they do for me? How did they enhance my life? Did they bring me joy? Who enjoyed them the most? Could they have been creating a disconnect on me fully receiving and/or giving love?

Why did I want implants?

The decision to get breast implants was completely my own. No one was talking me into getting them and no one was talking me out of getting them. After having baby number three I immediately wanted breast implants. I have always been obsessed with breasts. Let's face it, we are a breast-obsessed nation. Men love breasts but women are just as focused on them as our male counterpart. I was always comparing myself to the girls in the magazines, the models on TV, the women on the internet, the sexy blonde standing next to me in line at the supermarket and most of all I thought if I had nice, beautifully shaped, perfect breasts I would feel whole. I was searching for something outside of me to fix what I felt was broken. I started thinking if I had a perfect body then I know I would feel amazing all the time. To me, it seemed like the woman who looked more like playboy models had more joy and excitement in their life. They had more fun, they received more gifts and attention, they were more fun to be around and they received what I was looking for the most... love and acceptance. I was searching for a deep down desire to be fulfilled. The desire to feel 100 percent love in my heart. To awaken everyday not obsessed with my body. I thought that breast implants would solve this problem for me.

I thought my physical body was causing this disconnect. So on January 21st, 2006 I went under the knife. I choose, because of my lack of self-love, to be put to sleep then have my armpits cut open, a silicone bag was then inserted through this opening and 475CC of saline fluid was pumped inside those bags. The valves were then closed and my armpit was stitched up. I finally had the breasts that I had always dreamed of. They were full, round, lifted and so beautiful. I could stop being at war with my body.

I finally had super hooters. I secretly felt that big, nice breasts did have some supernatural power that I was craving. I grew up in a household of older boys and after hearing them speak often about girls I created this belief for myself. The belief was that girls with bigger breasts, were better... that was my own personal childhood interpretation. I started creating these beliefs about my physical body at such a young age. I was being controlled by my inner child. My inner little girl knew that having powerful breasts meant having control over all that I desired. I thought that super hooters would bring me love, acceptance and joy.

What did they do for me?

I did feel something awaken inside of me. It was the confidence of looking amazing in the clothes that I always dreamed of. I remember getting ready for a night out with my husband and I couldn't wait to put on that little black dress. It was short, to show off my sexy legs, it had an open back and tied around my neck but the most exciting part was it plunged down my neck line and opened up so very sensual to see my perfectly, not moving at all breasts. They were like a trophy that I was showing off to everyone. I was so excited to go out in this black dress of seduction. Wow, I was right, they were super hooters. They did have magical powers. They drew the attention from everyone. Men would glance, smile, stare in awe of these beautiful breasts and women would also glance, smile, sometimes glare and stare in awe of these beautiful breasts.

This was the power that I longed for. To have people admire and love me. To have the body that I have always wanted. To know what it feels like to have the perfect breasts. I had been wondering what this moment would feel like since I was a teenager. It was absolutely amazing. The outside attention was there, my body was looking fantastic, I looked great in all the clothes I wore. I should have been happy, loved, accepted and complete.

The first six months were great, but after that I reverted back to feeling disconnected and alone. Just like any new item we purchase, the newness wears off and my breast implants just weren't doing what I wanted them to do anymore. I no longer felt that cloud nine feeling. I still looked great and my breasts were still perfectly positioned and looking amazing but I had come crashing down from my breast implant high. They were still super hooters but I was no longer had access to their power. When I received my implants I was 29. Now I am 40. In this 10-year time frame I have expanded, contracted, blossomed, withered, grown, shrunk, loved, lost, awakened and healed. Having beautiful breasts is a true desire for most women. I always longed to look and feel super sexy and sensual. While having breast implants I noticed that it was not my breasts implants that did anything for me or I would have felt sensational the whole 10.5 years I had them. It was their ability to spark my inner confidence. That is why I call them super hooters. They had the ability to awaken my sensuality and my sexuality in a way that demanded attention even if I wasn't focused on getting attention. My breast implants awoke my deep sexual energy that I had forgotten was even there. This was the super hooter magic I was talking about.

During this 10.5 years of having two foreign objects in my body to enhance the look of my breasts I have learned a thing or two about myself. I am not my breasts. My breasts do not create happiness. My breasts are not the star of the show. My breasts are not what give me confidence. My breasts do not demand attention. I have breasts and they are part of my physical body but they do not define me. I get to choose how I view my breasts. I now choose to love them just as they are. They are soft, sensual, and perfectly imperfect. They are open to receiving love, passion, peace and pleasure.

Did they bring me joy?

Joy is found in the eye of the beholder. We choose to be in our joyous energy or we choose not to be. The way we look may shift that feeling momentarily but it will not transform our deepest beliefs about ourselves. Joy is our birthright and I thought that my breast would bring me more joy. I did feel joy after receiving them but it was superficial joy. It was fleeting joy. The joy I felt came on strong, lingered around for a while and then completely disappeared like the mountains in a dense fog. I know that the joy I felt was meant to be mine. I knew just like that mountain, it was still there, it is just covered with a thick layer of self-doubt and self-hatred. Our bodies can enhance the joy we have in our life but they do not activate joy on its own. Joy comes from within.

Who enjoyed them most?

I asked myself this question because I wanted to know if my breast implants were creating a disconnect in my ability to fully receive a beautiful connection inside my marriage. My husband is a very touchy guy (I truly am blessed that after 17 years together he still loves touching me) but when he would touch my breasts there was some running dialogue that sounded something like this. "He loves my breasts because they are huge and fake, He loves big boobs and I am so happy that I have these breasts implants, He is turned on by me because I have big breasts". This was something that ran in my brain sometimes, not all the time but it caused me some disdain for my husband. It was never his fault. He just wanted to enjoy my body and touch my breasts and to do that he had to caress the breast implant as well. So in a way my breast implants were creating a disconnect for me when it came to my husband caressing my breasts.

Sex in marriage is so important. I feel it is a relationship that we must cultivate and focus on. At first my breast implants brought more joy to the bedroom, but after a while they brought up even more self-doubt and activated my emotional pain. I experienced many different emotions and some of them were sadness, anger, guilt, shame, rejection and hatred. Sometimes I felt this way towards my husband and sometimes all these emotions were internalized. My sexuality was being compromised. I no longer felt that these were my breast. My implants started creating an energy that I was fake. My husband enjoyed my breast implants but he enjoys the energy of me more than my physical body. If I was feeling fake then there was no way I could show up in a feminine sensual space for him. He loved me with or without my breast implants and I finally realized that I would allow myself more healing and more self expression if I no longer had my breast implants. We both enjoyed them off and on but the time had come that my breast implants no longer were serving me. They were harming me.

How did they enhance my life?

When I was 29 and my breast implants were new and shiny, they enhanced my life. They enhanced it in a superficial way but it was definitely enhanced. I loved waking up and getting ready for the day. I enjoyed knowing that I could lay on my back and my breasts would stay perfectly positioned. I loved being playful with my husband and flashing him while I walked by never doubting that my breasts were in mint condition. I enjoyed wearing tight tops with no bra and I loved expressing my newfound feminine boobies!

After six months or so my breast implants were no longer enhancing my life. The emotional pain that I had once felt came back bearing gifts. My emotions were demanding to be felt, and for the first six months of having breast implants they were just laying back and waiting. They were allowing me to believe that all the pain I felt was due to my body not looking perfectly. Boy was I wrong. For the next six years I went on an emotional roller coaster that even the biggest lover of roller coasters would not enjoy. I gained 15 pounds so now I was no longer looking super hot anymore, as I gained all this weight in my mid section, so now I looked like a giant apple with big boobs. I felt sad, depressed, disconnected and alone. I was back at war with my body. After six years of this I thought I better do something different. It is not my physical body that is causing me unhappiness. It is my inner dialogue, my deep belief system and my inability to love myself completely.

The Healing Journey

I went on a healing journey. I discovered that awakening to the beauty of who I am at my core is what I was longing for. I wanted to feel amazing with or without this extra 15 pounds, with or without super hooters, with or without a successful business, and with or without perfection. I was looking for a deep, solid, passionate, and pleasurable relationship with myself. I was looking for self-acceptance and self-approval. I was searching for an understanding of the woman deep, down inside my soul. I know she was calling out to me like a siren in the night. She wanted to be seen, heard, felt and loved for the beautiful goddess she is. My breast implants did enhance my life. They played a huge part in me realizing that I am more than my physical appearance. I am more than my breasts. I am more than just a pretty face. I am more than my body. My breasts implants activated a deep desire to want to love myself for all that I am as well as love myself for all that I consider I am not. My breast implants spoke to my soul in a way that awoke a part of me that wanted to heal. The part of me that believed I was only worth how amazing my body looked. Most the time I didn't feel it looked amazing so I was always punishing myself. By getting breasts implants I found out that nothing I can do to my physical body will change the way I feel internally about myself. My belief systems that I created required some adjusting and that is the only thing that would allow me to feel like the sensual, sexy goddess that I truly am.

Could they have been creating a disconnect on me fully receiving and/or giving love?

Were they guarding my heart?

For me this was the most important and the deepest question I could ask myself. Did I get breast implants because I did not feel safe in the world and I wanted my heart to be protected? The answer to this didn't shock me. I knew the answer the moment I asked myself the question. I had breasts implants to protect my heart! The look was nice but the real, honest to goodness reason I got them was to guard my heart. My whole life I lived in some state of fear. I was born into fear and years later I still carried this childhood fear around with me. This fear was silent but it made its presence very clear all throughout my life. After having baby number three and feeling an intense fear about not being good enough, my subconscious did what it does best. It found a way to keep me feeling safe. When we don't feel safe in the world we usually find a way to assist us in feeling more at peace and ease. I choose to layer my heart. To put a protective covering over it so that my heart could remain hidden and free from pain. I had trapped my heart energy. It could no longer express itself in a complete way and I could no longer feel the essence of pure love. Through the ten and a half years that I had my breast implants I experienced a feeling of being in a glass prison cell.

I felt love and joy but it never felt pure, true and whole. It was always missing something. They kept me trapped inside so I could never fully express all the glitter and shine I had to offer. After receiving my breast implants I always felt like a part of me, a super powerful part of me was being suppressed. The breast implant layered my heart energy. I could no longer show up as 100 percent authentically me. I was now a woman who had her boobs done. I felt like a fake, a fraud and I felt as though I was trying to be something I was not .

Our heart is full of love energy. We give this energy and we receive this energy. When I had breast implants this energy was coming in and out of my heart through a very thick filter. I wanted to share my story, because my breast implants caused me to feel disconnected when it comes to a heart-to-heart connection. The implant is a solid object. Yes, breasts implants do have a bit of flexibility but when I would hug someone, the implant itself created resistance.

The Heart Path from Sexy Implants ~ Cameo Haag

I tried so many things to heal my heart and I know they all served me in deep and meaningful ways but the most importantly, the number one thing I did was get my breast implants removed. I can now feel a love that I knew was there but I could never fully grasp. I now feel a deep sense of gratitude when giving and receiving love. I can now feel a human to human connection when I give someone a hug. I can now wear cute tops and feel naturally beautiful. I now feel authentic in who I am as a woman and lover of my own perfectly imperfect breasts. My implants have been out for several months now and I know a part of me has awakened that I have been longing for. This may not be the case in every breast implant story but it was for me. So if you have breast implants or are thinking about getting them, ask yourself…

Do I really want my heart guarded by a security guard that I have no control over?

Am I willing to take the risks that are associated with breast implants for the rewards?

How are breast implants going to affect my life long term?

Why do I want breast implants?

Can I learn to just love my natural breasts for all they are?

Am I prepared to have surgery every 7-10 years, as this is the shelf life for breast implants?

Have I done research on both the positive and the negatives on getting breast implants?

Breast implants are a foreign object and our body will always feel a bit off when we are not living in our natural state of being. We are the divine feminine and when we create a decision that bigger or more perfect breasts will make us whole the universe will respond and awaken us to the truth of who we are. We are the receiving energy of love and light. We are the truth tellers and the lovers of life. We are the creators and the deliverers. We are the divine feminine full of soft, sensual, expanding energy. We are the women of the 21st century! We are not our breasts!

Cameo Haag

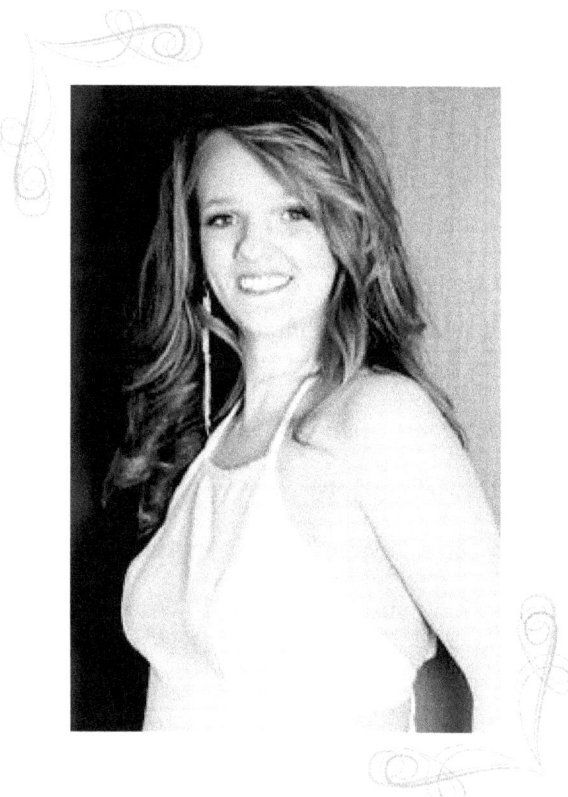

I am a mother of three, the wife of 1 and a lover of all things in life. I enjoy the good and the bad, the right and the wrong, the dark and the light, the love and the hate. I believe that we must know the sun to appreciate the moon. We must feel the sadness to experience the joy. I love expressing and feeling all my emotions and enjoy supporting others along their emotional journey as well. I am a licensed massage therapist and have been since 1996. I am certified in the emotion code, an

energy healing process, where we tap into old energies that may be blocking us from experiencing pleasure. I am a writer who blogs all about the power of releasing our heavy sexual energy and misbeliefs about sex so we can expand our yummy sexual creative energy and experience more peace, passion and pleasure in our life. I am a woman who has struggled with her body image every since I can remember. I am a woman who wants to be seen and remain hidden at the exact same time. I am a woman who knows she is a divine feminine goddess of love and light while simultaneously feeling that I am unworthy and no one could possible love me. I am a woman who wants to serve the world and show up powerfully but has these deep core beliefs that the world is not safe and no one will be there to receive me. I am a woman! I am the divine feminine who expresses herself openly and honestly and knows that the world deserves more love. I love you and want to express my appreciation for you taking the time to read my story. Please reach out to me on facebook or on my blog at www.sexlessmarriagenomore.com.

CHAPTER 3
WELL, I NEVER…
Leslie Lang

Wearing an oversized hospital gown with the ties in the front, I wait for my doctor in the chilly, sterile room. I wonder how many other people have worn this hospital gown before me… Ew. My eyes wonder around, noting the health-related posters on the walls and the stacks of pamphlets with advice about avoiding the flu and other common illnesses. The paper under my butt crinkles and rips as I shift to make sure my gown is covering as much of body as possible. I glance down at my feet and realize that a pedicure is way overdue. I hear the doctor grab my file from the pocket mounted to the outside of the door. I flinch back to reality. Yes, I requested a woman doctor. Who else understands breasts more than a doctor who actually has them? The doctor's eyes are kind and her smile, genuine. She introduces herself to me and asks how I am… "I don't know how I am… I was hoping you did," I respond with light sarcasm. The doctor takes a deep breath and says, "You have breast cancer and it is invasive." "I'll say!" I respond with medium sarcasm. She explains that because of my young age of 39, she suggests breast surgery to remove the cancer, then chemotherapy, and then radiation. "Wow, doctor… How skinny will I get during this?" I ask, with a slightly, hopeful smile. Actually, I am prescribing you steroids, which will actually make you gain a lot of weight during the treatment process. I shake my head and yell "FUCKING CANCER!" What the fuck!?!? I have breast cancer??? How dare anyone even put the ugly word, "cancer" with the lovely word, "breast!" That seems criminal. What did I do or not do to deserve this? I run through a list of my sins in my head. Hmm… There are some bad ones in there, but not enough to warrant this kind of punishment.

I never thought that I'd ever get a "boob job." The surgeon explains the difference between a lumpectomy and a mastectomy. Remove part of my breast or all of my breast. I couldn't imagine having one large breast completely removed and the other large breast still there. How could I walk in a straight line? How would my shirts fit? I love my nipples and didn't want to be so lopsided, so I decided to get a lumpectomy. You can always remove more breast tissue later, if necessary, I thought. After the lumpectomy surgery was completed, the surgeon told me that she almost had to remove the whole breast, because of the location on the cancer. Still groggy from the anesthesia, I ask about my nipples. "Did you save my nipples!?!?" Thank goodness the answer was "yes."

I never thought that I'd ever get any tattoos. But, now, I have three. They are blue tattooed dots around my left breast. I guess that's better than a faded, unrecognizable dolphin or hummingbird tattoo in my bikini area. The table is cold on my bare back as a huge machine is lowered just above my chest. Three nurses work together to properly align the machine in between my newly inked, tiny tattoos.

I'm scared. How the hell did I get here? I feel like I'm part of an alien experiment. I thank the nurses and ask them to stay with me during my radiation treatment. One nurse smiles kindly and says that the nurses can't be in the room during the radiation sessions. As the nurses were leaving, but before they closed what looked to be an 18" thick, steel door, I yell, "Wait a minute, is this thing dangerous?!?!?!?" The heavy door slams shut and over the intercom, I'm instructed to stay still and hold my breath. The radiation machine was quiet and seemed harmless. However, I saw the results a few days later. My breast was badly burned and required several applications of cooling lotion throughout the days. There's a completely separate building for the radiation treatments. In the waiting room, I see women, wearing wigs, hats or scarves, working on puzzles. I've been sentenced to 30 doses of radiation, so I might as well help put those puzzles together. I scan the room and try to figure out who these women are and why they are here. Among the older women who've had plenty of time to get cancer, there's a young mother, only 31 years old. Over several weeks of treatment, I get to know these ladies, as we cross paths at the same time, every day. I make a poster with all of our names and boxes to check after every one of our radiation treatments. We finished all of the many puzzles that were in the waiting room. I tried to not let it bother me that there were a couple of pieces missing from most of them. We celebrated after the poster was fully checked off.

I never thought that I'd ever have to know what an oncologist is, let alone, need one. I take the elevator to the fourth floor and walk to the oncology department. I check in at the front desk and the woman puts my file on the stack behind her. I scan the waiting room for the other unlucky people touched by cancer. I can see people in the different stages of chemo…some with hair…some without. They all look tired and worried, and with good reason. A nurse soon summons me to the back, where she weighs me and takes my blood pressure. I'm scared. Of course, my blood pressure will be high…I'm in the hospital, waiting to be injected with poison. I'm transferred to a large chair with a rolling IV drip at my side. The nurse, wearing colorful and cheerful scrubs, gently punctures my upper chest, where the surgeon had inserted a port. This makes the chemo administration a lot easier to start. The doctor explained the type of chemo I would be getting, however, all I heard was the teacher from the Snoopy cartoons. I think one part of the chemo was mustard seed, sometimes used in bombs and the dregs from the bottom of the sea…OK, I didn't know exactly what it was and I guess it really didn't matter, because I didn't have any other ideas. I actually consented to have poison injected into my body, in hopes that it would kill the cancer cells. My body seems OK after the first treatment. I thought it would be much worse than this. I can handle this. Little did I know that the chemo has a cumulative effect. I got sicker with each treatment. After two chemo treatments, I'm at my office and overhear two coworkers talking about me. One guy asks the other guy how I'm doing… The other guy, who's desk is next to mine, responds that he's afraid to ask…because (in a loud whisper) "She's got bbbreast cancer." I interrupt their conversation and ask, would you be more comfortable if we call it "breastical" cancer? How about "chestical" cancer? I get it, you guys, it doesn't make sense to have the word for a lovely body part next to the horrible word, cancer. But, please don't treat me any differently; I'll still kick your ass in sales, with or without hair. With both hands, I grab clumps of my hair and throw it at them. They are speechless…and scared. I laugh out loud and continue down the hall.

I never thought that I'd ever be bald. My hair starting falling out after the second chemo treatment. My hair stylist colored a streak of my remaining hair, hot pink. It was my last-ditch effort to have some control. My head soon looked like that of a baby bird with patches and whiffs of hair here and there. It was time. Time to accept my inevitable baldness. My dear friends came over and helped me shave my head. In anticipation of losing my hair after my chemo treatments, I bought three expensive, natural-looking wigs. I want to look good, if I'm going to do this cancer thing. My bald head is cold. While wearing my natural-looking wigs and interacting with people, I realize that I'm always worried about if they know that I'm wearing a wig… Is it obvious? Is it lop-sided on my head? Do they know that I have cancer? Would it matter if I did? I felt like I had to combat all of that by telling them about the wig, before it got too distracting. So, I decided to wear wigs that were obviously wigs. Purple, pink, teal, and blue… In an attempt to "cheer" me up, some ladies would say how neat it would be to wear fun, colorful wigs… Well, get cancer and find out, I think to myself. It's one thing to be bald and wearing a wig, out of necessity, and it's another to be wearing a festive wig to a party. I hold back my thoughts, because I know that these women are only trying to help and don't really know what to say.

Well, I NEVER... ~ Leslie Lang

I never thought that I'd be like a Barbie doll... down there. At lunch with a girlfriend, I excuse myself to go to the bathroom. As usual, I hover over the toilet and pee. I feel the warm pee flow down my leg and into my high heel shoe and onto the floor. I panic, stand up, and see the big mess I've made. I scramble for enough toilet paper and seat covers to soak it all up... When I return to the table, I tell my friend about my bathroom blooper and suggest that we leave immediately. "You've never had a Brazilian bikini wax?!??," she asked. "No. No, I haven't," I responded. Apparently, without hair down there, I need to point my little "bean" downward so the pee flows into the toilet and not down my leg. Lesson learned.

I never thought that I'd ever be so vulnerable... I'm not a person to ask anyone for help and I'm a recovering control freak. Getting this diagnosis really made me want to get something off my chest–Cancer. And I can't do that alone. My mouth is dry and tastes like the inside of a gym locker. I can only eat popsicles. My nausea is overwhelming. My body aches and I just want to curl up and cry. Cards, calls, gifts, and visits...people came out of the woodwork to help me, any way they could. They cooked and cleaned for me... They did my laundry and grocery shopping for me... They brought over funny movies, cannabis cookies and magic potions... Eileen, my long-time friend, came up from LA to help me get through my lumpectomy surgery and rehabilitation. She came with soft pajamas with buttoned-up fronts to easily access my scars, and a portable DVD player for my long chemotherapy sessions. I was humbled by all of the loving support, company, and gifts... truly humbled.

I never thought that I'd ever be a professional stand-up comedian. In order to flush the remaining chemo out of my body, I attended a well-respected healing center in Southern California. At the end of the grueling three-week regimen, I participated in the center's talent show, as the hostess. Apparently, I was hilarious and people thought that I performed comedy professionally. Three people, from "The Biz" pulled me aside after the talent show and insisted that I pursue a career in comedy. You're a natural! They said. You should have your own show, they said. Then, they double-dog-dared me to perform at an open mic at my local Improv when I returned home to San Jose. I took that dare and that's how it all got started! Holy shit, I love the stage and spotlight! Who knew that a terrible disease would springboard me into what is now my big passion? Joking about my breast cancer on stage is cathartic for me and allows others to see the lighter side of cancer. So, I was 40, fat, bald, with only 1.75 breasts. Guys used to say that I had a "nice rack." Now I have more of a half rack, but still nice. My doctor told me that my good sense of humor and positive attitude may have helped me heal faster than most. I looked at the doctor, pointed at my left bra cup and said, "When I see this cup, I see it as half FULL." I was determined to still do the things I enjoy, despite having two different sized breasts, so I entered a wet T-shirt contest. I came in 1st and 3rd.

I never thought that I'd ever say that breast cancer was one of the best things that has happened to me… I had cancer, but cancer did not have me. I experienced and learned so much along the journey. I learned how to surrender and let people help me. I was humbled by all of the love and support I received. I got out of a toxic marriage. I changed my priorities. I performed stand-up comedy at clubs, fundraisers, and private parties. I surround myself with positive and kind people. I only work with nice people. I have fun and laugh a lot. I don't worry about the small stuff… because after surviving cancer, it's ALL small stuff.

Leslie Lang

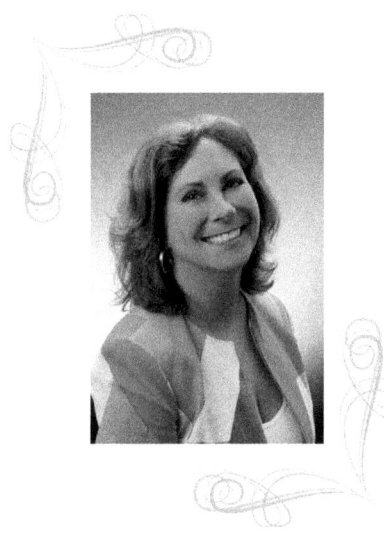

Leslie Lang *has been an enthusiastic and successful Realtor® with Keller Williams Realty-Silicon Valley for the last 12 years. She enjoys putting a fun and creative spin on home-buying and selling, using videos, props and clever communications. Surviving breast cancer in 2007 was the catalyst she needed to share her funny thoughts on stage as a stand-up comedienne. Performing stand-up comedy is cathartic and counterbalances the gravity associated with most real estate transactions. Leslie loves to use her real estate knowledge and sense of humor to have her clients laughing all the way to the bank.*

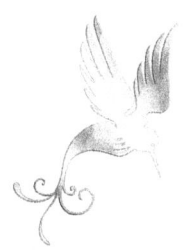

CHAPTER 4
BREASTS: THE KEY TO FEMININE VITALITY

Dr. Kim D'Eramo

Do you love your breasts?

*Y*ou may have never been asked this by a doctor, but it happens that as a woman, the way you *feel* about your body is one of the most important factors that contributes to your health.

From a functional standpoint, breasts are used to nurture our young, or to receive tenderness from a lover, increasing oxytocin levels and giving us a sense of connection and bonding, while from a societal standpoint, they represent so much more.

A sign of womanhood and our sexuality, there are many ideas and judgments about how breasts should look, how they should feel, what size they should be, and whether we should enlarge them or have them surgically removed.

Breasts are objectified, lauded, praised, celebrated, worshipped, feared, criticized, manipulated,... and they are *sacred*.

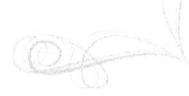

No other body part receives so much attention and scrutiny.

Our breasts represent the way we care for and nurture others and also have to do with the way we nurture ourselves. For many women, after years of nurturing and caring for family, parents, and community, breast disease develops and they are finally forced to put themselves first. For the first time, they *must* prioritize their needs or they quite simply could die. When we sacrifice and compromise ourselves for others, putting their needs before our own, our body suffers.

We're in a culture that trains women to put others first. When we want to be happier, we do more for others and give more of ourselves, looking for self-worth and personal fulfillment. Often when I ask women *"What do you really want?"* they simply don't know. *"I've never considered what I want, since I've been so focused on caring for everyone else"* is the most common answer. Women often feel guilty putting their needs first or asking for assistance, as if somehow that makes them inadequate or selfish. We overtax ourselves, constantly putting energy into meeting the needs of others, while ignoring our own. This directly affects the part of us designed to nurture others: our breasts.

Dis-ease with our breasts applies not only with mothers and adult women, but even in the very young. Girls who develop breasts early may attract undesired sexual attention, while girls who are delayed in breast development may feel inadequate. There is often shame with having larger-than-average breasts at an early age, and young girls either hide their bodies or flaunt them as a way to deal with insecurity. Currently, women and girls are not given much guidance in how to release shame about their bodies, and embody their breasts with confidence and deep respect for their femininity. We simply aren't taught how to handle this power. This is part of what I'm here to change in my practice of MindBody Medicine.

I've seen many women develop back and neck pain by subconsciously hiding their femininity and literally, trying to hide their body. They feel self-conscious, insecure, and even threatened by the world around them, so they try to make themselves smaller to diminish the risk of being seen and allow them to disappear into the background. They crouch, slouch, and hunch to diminish attention on their breasts and their beauty, out of fear, shame, or self-denial. When this type of "hiding" begins at a young age, it can result in scoliosis, hunchback deformity, chronic pain, and even chronic depression.

When young women develop breasts without being properly initiated into womanhood, guided and assisted by women who *have* integrated a strong sense of self-worth, security, confidence, and self-love, this is especially difficult. The body begins to change and express emotions, physical signals, and chemical signals that enhance sexuality, attraction, attractiveness, and maturity that they simply are not prepared to handle. This often brings a sense of shame, as though sexuality is wrong and should be hidden. Many young girls carry this throughout their adulthood and never have an outlet to release this self-judgment and poor body-image. It affects diet and nutrition, fitness, sexuality, and even the confidence we have to enter a career with confidence.

We're also in a culture where femininity is seen as inferior and weak. There is a big misunderstanding about the true essence of femininity and it's often seen as subordinate and subservient to the masculine. We're bombarded with messages to literally stay small physically, and with it, there is the message that we are less-than societally. No wonder so many women have poor body image and eating disorders. We've simply not been shown how to honor the power that lies within our bodies!

The feminine essence is about stillness, receiving, softness, being, creativity, cyclic change, and the *unseen power* within. We've been living in a world that primarily honors and values the masculine essence: action, achievement, exertion, overcoming, and *external power*, so when there's the call of the body to step into the feminine essence, most women resist this, and reject themselves. Nowhere is this more overt than with the breasts, the most uniquely feminine expression of our bodies.

The masculine essence is about linear, unchanging steadiness, the ability to hold a constant foundation for the ever-changing flowing feminine. We all have masculine and feminine energies within us. Typically, women have more feminine than masculine energy. There is meant to be a balance and harmony here. When women are conditioned to embody only their masculine attributes, it goes against their nature. Menstruation becomes a "curse" and the body literally generates hormones and chemicals that tense muscles, restrict blood flow, and make it painful and depressing to go through their monthly cycle.

The body is constantly listening to and reflecting our ideas about it.

Women's bodies are the ever-changing vessel of Life, literally, the space through which new life flows. When they're pushed, restricted, judged, and held to rigid expectations and demands, they cannot function normally. Life flow is restricted, and disease follows on every level: physically, mentally, and emotionally.

Whether or not there is a medical diagnosis of premenstrual syndrome (PMS), polycystic ovarian syndrome (PCOS), anxiety/depression, endometriosis, uterine fibroids, fibrocystic breast disease, or even breast cancer, when there is dis-ease with your feminine essence, there will be some level of physical disease in your body. There cannot NOT be. The physical body is impacted by every thought and belief we have about ourselves, our womanhood, and our feminine power, even if it's just a lack of understanding of what that really is.

When we think our power lies in our achievements, our worth seems to come from outside of ourselves. We must constantly work harder and harder to *prove* to ourselves and others that we are worthy of love. The cellular messages in our body reflect this discord. Cortisol, stress hormone, levels rise and stay high throughout the day. Inflammatory chemicals flood the body. These changes are not only associated with anxiety, overweight, chronic fatigue, autoimmune disease, depression, and diabetes, but they're also known to ignite the cellular changes that cause cancer to develop. This has been shown to even affect our DNA expression. That means if you have the genes for breast cancer, these chemical reactions activate them.

Likewise, when we live in harmony and balance with our body, embracing our femininity and allowing it to be expressed in healthy ways, this *decreases* cortisol, inflammatory hormones, brings physical wellbeing, and turns "*off*" the genes that cause breast cancer. That means even if you *do* have the genes for breast cancer, you can keep your breasts and remain cancer free.

The disconnection with our feminine essence and lack of harmony in the body prevents us from tapping into our body's wisdom and guidance. It causes fear, anxiety, and a lack of awareness about what choices contribute to our health. We do not need to live in this discord and distress, constantly seeking out answers from experts, books, or the latest research in health science. There is so much Wisdom in our bodies when we're in harmony with our feminine essence! This opens up awareness that guides us in everything from what foods to eat for ideal health, to which relationship to choose for an ideal partnership, to which career will bring the greatest prosperity. Our internal guidance assists us with our overall health, abundance, and balance in all areas of life.

When we're disconnected with our bodies due to this self-rejection, we cut off this wisdom, calling on the *mind* to figure out the answers to everything. There is now a billion-dollar industry to tell us what to eat, how to have a great relationship and how be fit and slim, and *still* we're more overweight, lonely, and sick than any culture ever before in history.

With the excess of masculine energy, we assert ourselves, overwork, over think, push too hard, and strive for more, instead of opening, allowing, and receiving. This creates illness in the body, discord in relationships, and lack of passion in our work.

Here is an example of what this looks like:

Ann was a medical student who worked hard and push herself to succeed. Because she'd been raised in a conventional family, she learned that her worth had to do with her achievements. She had seen her mother suffer rejection from her father, and stay in the marriage because she was dependent on him financially. Ann vowed she would never let that happen to her. She prioritized work and her studies, and although she had a relationship with a man she loved, her first priority was her career.

During medical school, Ann developed fatigue and began to gain weight. Previously slim and fit, she began to feel *out of control* of her body and her weight. She used running to stay fit, and pushed herself to run even when she didn't feel like running. Her body wore down from injuries, overuse, and pain. She used pain medication, but more problems and illness developed and Ann continued to feel like her body was falling apart. Eventually, her doctor found that her thyroid labs were abnormal and told her she had hypothyroid disease.

That is when Ann decided to surrender. She knew her body could heal, and although she had no idea what to do, she reached out for assistance from me. What we found was Ann's fear of failure and need to excel had depleted her body out. There was also struggle in her relationship. Because Ann was adamantly against being dependent on a man, she subconsciously withdrew from her boyfriend, which created turmoil and distress in the relationship.

Through Skype and phone sessions together, we rebalanced Ann's body, and released the fear keeping her from surrendering, receiving, and allowing. Her body healed. Her fatigue resolved and her energy returned. She lost weight and was free from pain. When she returned to her doctor, her thyroid had returned to normal. She no longer required medications.

There is so much power in integrating a healthy feminine essence and allowing the flow of health. This has to do not only with our cellular and hormone balance, but also the choices we make in our lives. If you've ever had a day when you just don't feel like working, but kept pushing, only to become fatigued and unable to perform, you know what it's like to have too much masculine energy. We strive to get ahead and miss the signals from our body telling us to slow down and receive. We simply don't value that *receiving* could contribute more to us than doing.

Many women live this way and opt for a more masculine expression of power, productivity, and outer action. We've been conditioned to deny the signals from the feminine essence, which are more based on the inner, unseen power than outer action and productivity. It's not seen, so we think it doesn't matter. We undervalue our innate value, and our world reflects that.

For many women with premenstrual syndrome, hormone imbalance, pelvic disease, and breast disease, there is imbalance with these masculine and feminine energies. The way they feel about their body is registered physically and creates disharmony and disease.

How do you know if you have an imbalance in your masculine/feminine energies?

How you *feel* about your breasts will tell you a LOT about how this masculine/feminine balance.

Take a look at your breasts naked in the mirror.

How do you feel when you look at them?

Is there an internal dialogue you're aware of?

Are they too saggy?...

Not large enough?...

Too large?...

Ugly?...

Do you feel embarrassed when you look at yourself naked?

Maybe there's just a feeling of discomfort, or even disgust.

Notice this! It is valuable feedback about the messages you're sending to your body, specifically the feminine parts.

Here's an exercise to find out how you really feel about expressing your feminine self.

- Stand tall.
- Jut out your chest and hold your shoulders back.
- Let your head fall back and shout out to the world: "*I'm a woman! Take me fully and completely!*"

This is what the feminine energy does. It *surrenders* to the masculine.

The inner feminine power surrenders to the outer masculine world.

Does this make you feel diminished? Subordinate? Threatened?

That's how you've been trained to view femininity.

Does it make you feel good? Exhilarated? Sexy? Excited? *Divine?*

That's an indication that you're balanced in your feminine expression.

In today's world where there has been so much focus on the masculine, where we've been conditioned to work hard, learn more, and achieve, we want to be in *control* instead of surrendering to a higher Wisdom. We set goals, assert ourselves, and push to get what we want. This is the opposite of what the feminine energy has for us. It gets translated in our bodies.

The feminine aspect moves us to surrender, release, and allow instead of force. This allows us to receive so much more! When we suppress this natural flow, we hold on tightly to our goals and agenda, exhaust our body, and block the ease, joy, and freedom we most deeply desire.

Years ago, when I developed an autoimmune illness, I was brought face to face with this imbalance within myself. I had worked hard for years to get into medical school, and was studying, running regularly, eating healthy, and pretty regimented in my life.

I got up early to work out, attended classes all day, then studied hard all evening. When I was exhausted, I would take a nap, but then go for a run to turn myself back "on" and keep going. As the illness set in: joint pain, muscle spasm, severe fatigue, weight gain and bloating, I would push myself to overcome the symptoms. I understood "mind-over-matter" and tried hard to overcome the illness.

I believed that if I surrendered to my body, things would get worse.

After trying multiple medications and therapies, my illness was worse after a year. I would have intermittent flu-like symptoms where I could no longer run, and sometimes took pain medications to get through the day.

Finally, I was diagnosed with a rare form of late-onset juvenile rheumatoid arthritis and told I would require multiple medications to calm the flare up in my immune system. I would have to live without rugs and curtains, use special kinds of detergents and cleaning solutions, and would no longer be able to run.

I was devastated to learn of this diagnosis and nearly broke down in tears, right there in the Harvard-trained doctor's office... until I remembered that *I didn't believe in this way of treating the body*. I didn't believe my body was broken and could not heal. I didn't believe this was just the way things were and I would have to deal with it.

The next day I developed a new relationship with my body. When I felt my symptoms, instead of trying to overcome them, fix them, or figure them out, I simply sat with them, stayed present to my body and asked what it needed from me. "*Slow down*" was the answer and "*relax*." I listened more and more closely and I followed. There was no longer the fear that things would get worse if I surrendered, or the idea that I was a victim to this illness and it was hopeless. Instead I allowed my body to teach me and guide me. I surrendered my agenda and was open to receive something new. It changed me for life.

I became comfortable with my body, my cyclic, changing nature, and began to accept it instead of trying to conquer it. When there was pain, I would relax and send my body love. When there was fatigue, I would simply *relax my body instead of fighting it*. I trusted and allowed the power within me to do what it needed to do. This changed everything! Within 10 days I was symptom-free and my body had completely healed.

I relaxed my body and allowed the power within me to do what it needed to do.

As soon as my body received what it needed, it easily restored balance and health. I stopped fearing my body and started loving and accepting it instead. This inner relationship of *ease, receiving, and allowing* is part of our feminine energy and is deeply needed in so many of us.

Loving our breasts is the ultimate expression of this Divine Feminine power. When we allow our feminine expression of beauty, *as we are*, without fear, we allow the flow of nature through our body and life. This is powerfully healing.

I've created tools to assist you with developing a positive body image. Whether you feel shame sexually, are insecure about your body or your breasts, are afraid of being feminine and sexual, or you've developed disease and are not clear on what to do, connecting in Love with your body is the key to inviting healing.

At www.DrKimD.com/breastbook you will find resources for releasing shame, abuse, and a negative body image so that you easily embody your feminine form with grace and ease. These MindBody tools not only change the way you *feel* about your body, they also generate healthy chemical changes shown to reverse pain, inflammation, overweight, Use these tools to assist your body with living at ideal weight and fitness and to give you that beautiful glow of a confident, secure, loving woman.

I look forward to connecting with you and hearing about what majesty awakens within you through using these tools!

As women, we are goddesses, here to love and nurture ourselves so that we can love and nurture this world. Unlock your inner goddess power proudly and shine your light. Honoring yourself and prioritizing your needs is the *greatest* gift you can bring to the world.

Dr. Kim D'Eramo

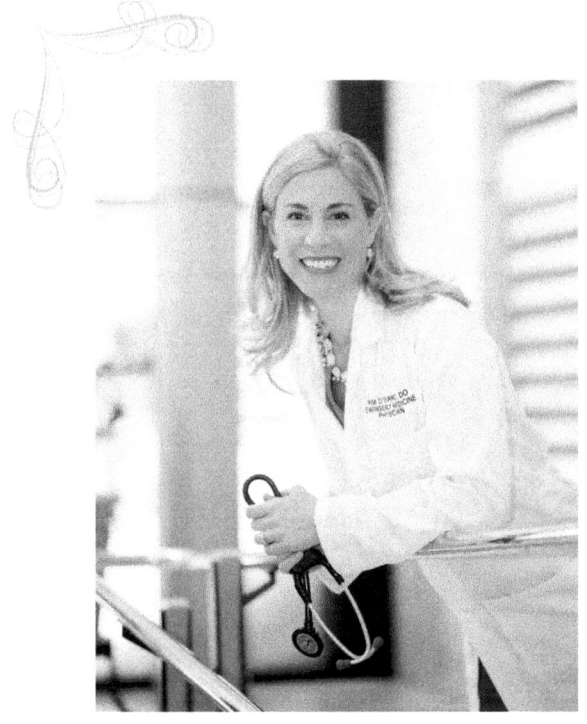

Dr. Kim D'Eramo *is a physician and bestselling author of* The MindBody Toolkit. *After healing herself from an autoimmune illness doctors said would be life-long, she created a medical practice centered around activating the body's ability to heal. She has now assisted thousands in living pain-free, anxiety-free, and reversing chronic illness and fatigue without medications. Dr. Kim started The American Institute of Mind Body Medicine to share with other doctors and wellness practitioners, how to "Be the Medicine" that heals your patients.*

You can find Dr. Kim at www.DrKimD.com.

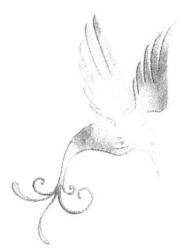

CHAPTER 5
HAVING RICH BREASTS IS AN HONOR

Nicole Richardson

There is no secret that my mother and I hold a special bond since birth, through breasts. Being the only girl of four, my parents have always wanted the best for their daughter. From the start, I was given the best nutrients and care while being breast fed by my mother. As I grew older, our bond became stronger while spending quality time together, having an open line of communication and given comfort and encouragement while participating in personal activities and creating innovative ideas is when I knew that having rich breasts is an honor.

Spending Quality Time

Growing up, my mother was always busy singing and hosting our parent's gospel radio and television show, but she would schedule a date and time a time to spend with her only daughter. I personally knew how important our relationship was and the bond we shared. Each and every Monday was mother and daughter time. My mom formed

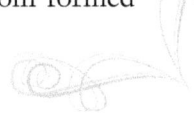

a group called Jo's girls. In this group was all of my girl cousins that were around the same age as I was. It was like my mom was not only a parent, she had also became a mentor as well. On each Monday, we would plan a pickup location for all the girls and ride to the mall. The mall was the best place for us teenagers. We would have dinner, meet other teenagers and shop until we dropped. I began to notice as a teen, the structure of my body was changing.

On Monday nights, we would drive 30 miles outside of my small home town to shop for everything I needed. Most importantly, for me, was shopping for bras at this particular time. My hometown only had a few shopping centers and we had to travel far to the nearest mall. I love to shop for shoes and clothes but I really needed the proper bra size. I would go up and down in sizes. I remember going to one particular brand name store and getting sized. I chose this store because it would have a wide variety of colors with a nice selection of bras and trained fitters. Early during the week was the best time to get bra accessories too. I was thin and trim so it was much easier for me to find a nice bra for my breasts. To others, bras can sometimes be the hardest thing to find. For some reason, my mother always knew the correct size and what bra was best for me. It was like my mom had super powers or something. She would always know the exact size I needed. I would always want big breasts like everyone else so once I picked out my colorful artistic bra, I would stuff it with tissue pushing them up as if my chest was bigger. I do not know why I did this, but I can tell you it was so much fun. My brothers thought I was crazy. I really miss those days. It was extremely nice creating memories and having so much fun spending time together with my mother.

Open Communication

In my life, having lines of open communication is very important. It is key and dear to my heart and something special that my mom and I both share in our mother and daughter relationship. My mother is the truth and speaks nothing but the truth. She does not hold back anything and this why I love her.

As I have grown in to a young woman, my body has changed from thin to thick. I am no longer that little skinny cheerleader on the football field. My college days in South Carolina got the best of me. Late nights studying, and just grabbing a quick snack to eat at crazy times. Having those unlimited chicken and Philly cheese steaks being that I was not on any set schedule. I gained weight. Immediately my mother noticed. She is very open about letting me know that things are getting out of hand. I would notice a change in my growth as well as my breasts. When I would lose weight, my breasts would shrink. My body does its own thing from time to time, I would go up and down and still do.

I could call up my mother anytime on the phone to share openly that my breasts were increasing in size along with my weight. A mother wants the best for her child. She would always instill in me on having good health, and informing me on the importance getting a regular checkup. In my family, there was a list of health problems on both sides and I knew my mom was concerned on passing anything down in our immediate family. She openly communicates with me to exercise, eat properly and pray. She would also give me the best advice on checking body at home to ensure that my body is okay through self-exams. I didn't know a lot about self-exams, so I would go and research on the web on how do just that.

While at home, I was told by my mother to look in the mirror observe and check out my body starting with my breasts, feel around your breast and the nipple area for any lumps, dimples or soreness. If I do feel something different or out of order, then inform her so that she could make an appointment to take me to the doctor immediately.

My mother was there to protect me and ensure that I was never too young or too old understand that no matter what the subject at hand was. I would notice during my menstrual cycle that my breasts would become more tender and sore. I try to change my diet. I work out and use less salt. I feel this helps with my breasts. Often times, I reduce the time I spend wearing a bra, becomes sometimes I just want to let loose and be free.

I know it is not easy for me to be as open as I can be but I am well aware that my mom is my confidante. I can confide in her like she can confide in with me. It truly feels good to have my mom as a confidante. Our experience together is an unbreakable bond, our relationship is strong I consider my mother a friend as well.

Comfort and Encouragement

I can remember at a very young age my mother comforting and encouraging me to be the best and do my best while participating in activities. My parents were very active in the community and they also ensured that my brothers and I were involved in some activity. The activities that we were involved in was not just any activity it was an activity where we could be innovative creating our own ideas.

One of the activities I will never forget and that stood out to me the most in regards to having rich breasts as an honor was The Miss South Carolina Teen USA Pageant 1996. While in high school, I was a contestant in the Miss South Carolina Teen USA Pageant and sometimes I still cannot believe it.

One of the key elements in determining what to wear was knowing your body proportions. For example, Are you full figured? Are your breasts flat? This was just a few of the questions to was key to have answers to in determining the proper pageant wear. I know that when walking, you have to stand straight walk with a poise, but do your shoulders and breasts balance out? Your overall look is important when it comes to body proportions. There was information given by the pageant officials to the contestants to seek help in body contouring from the professionals if the contestants wanted to have a perfect look during the pageant. While participating as a contestant we ask to wear three selected interview outfits such as: a bathing suit, business suit and a pageant gown.

My body type was growing from thin to thick. My thighs had gotten thick, my buttocks were getting bigger and my breasts well let us just say they were forming and getting plump. As a contestant, I not only wanted to look good but also have nice pageant wear that was pleasing to my parents and myself. My father is a minister so I still wanted to not show too much skin or have too much breasts out and still accomplish my goal in winning my first major pageant without having an outfit that looked a little too risqué. Looking fabulous was important and image is everything especially on this special day.

While preparing for this particular pageant, my mother and I were always bonding as we did since I was born. She was taking me shopping, asking me what did I like, what color material did I want to use. We just found it a little challenging when looking for the proper fit clothing because of my breasts and body proportion and size. My mother never knew this but, I was embarrassed because of my body and breasts. I had a low self-esteem issue because I didn't want anyone to say anything about my changes it was like my breasts had grew over night.

As I mentioned earlier during my teen years my body was changing as I was growing. Sometimes it could get a little discouraging looking at the other teens. In comparison to the contestants that were partaking in the pageant from the headshots, I could see that some of the other girls were very different. Different in color, shape and sizes some of them was tall, slim or flat chested verses others thicker with a heavier size breasts but still small. I also even noticed that some girls received implants. The great thing is that we are all different and unique in our own light. I was just having a hard time shopping and getting my outfits together. The more and more I would shop for pageant wear, it was the more and more that I realized the importance of having the proper shapewear and undergarments.

I was beginning to get frustrated as I went to the different boutique shops and stores. I began reflecting and thinking what should I do. Then I realized that I wanted to stand out and do something different.

I Quit Looking in Stores

I quit looking in the stores! I remembered that I had a very creative and talented aunt that could make anything from scratch. My aunt was so awesome she made all of her niece's gowns during the prom seasons and graduations. The thinking cap in my head went off and I thought it would be a great idea to have her join in on this project with us since she could make clothes. I asked my mother because she is so comforting and encouraging in anything that I would do. She also thought that it was a great idea. Fast forwarding, my aunt took all my measurements from the bust line to the waist line. My family did not want me to have my breasts all out in the bathing suits or pageant gown. My aunt began to sew and put all my outfits together. I was so excited. I was just hoping that everything would fit just right. It was time for the pageant, I tried on all of my outfits. I must say I loved them. My breasts fit perfectly in all three outfits. That was my major concern. I looked so pretty. I really enjoyed participating in the Miss South Carolina Teen USA Pageant in 1996. I was just so happy to have the comfort, support and encouragement of my family.

Conclusion

We all come in different shapes and different sizes it is an honor to have rich breasts. I've had some great experiences with my mother and bonding since birth. Our bond became stronger while spending quality time together, having an open line of communication and given comfort and encouragement while participating in personal activities and creating innovative ideas.

NICOLE RICHARDSON

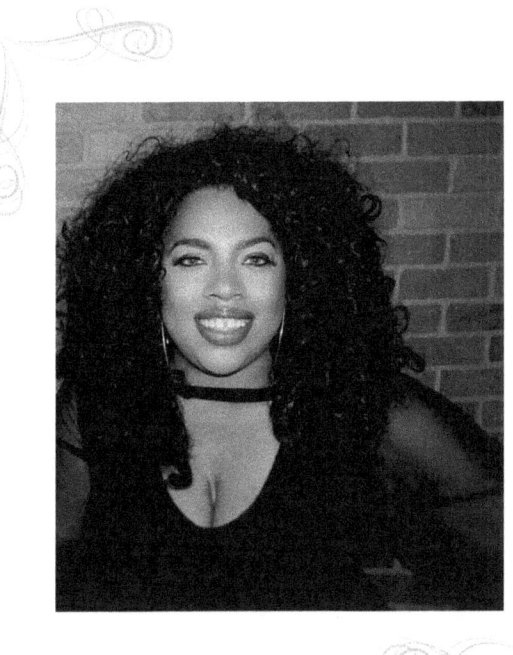

Nicole Richardson, *aka Nikki Rich, is the CEO of The Nikki Rich Show, an Award-Winning Television and Radio Show Network that is based out of Los Angeles, CA. Nikki is also currently an OWN Ambassador of the OWN: Oprah Winfrey Network. She interviews with her show Live at The Oprah Winfrey Network the Cast of the The OWN TV Shows, and the official Media for Oprah Life You Want Tour, Super Soul Sessions 1 and 2.*

CHAPTER 6
BYE BYE BRA, HELLO FREEDOM!

Elisabeth Schweiger

I gave up wearing a bra. That's right. Months ago, after years of soul-searching, I decided there was more to who I am than the sum of how my breasts looked in a shirt. That may sound funny to some, but it has been a lifelong journey of presenting my body for the enjoyment of others in order to feel good about myself.

One day early on in this newfound freedom, I put a bra on for a few hours while I was running errands. My body cried out in pain the entire time. As soon as I got back home, the bra came off, and my body cried again, but this time it was out of pure elation! Needless to say, the bra hasn't graced my body since.

I'm assuming many are wondering how I got to a place where I could actually choose to liberate myself from one of our society's most stringent social norms. Let's be serious; choosing to go braless, in public especially, is such a taboo! My story is a complicated plot with many details, but I will try to focus on the most important parts. I predict these words will resonate with many women. One of the greatest challenges

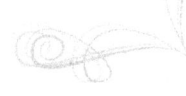

faced by our culture in this day and age is the struggle to be perfect for the pleasure of others. Males and females alike are impacted greatly by demands such as these. My intentions for telling my story are personally motivated. I know I must come face-to-face with my demons and put them into the light, for them to be conquered. However, I am also grateful to know that reading my story might inspire others to begin listening to and honoring their bodies, as well. So, here I am as I bare my soul; naked before you, as I describe my relationship with my body.

I was 10 years old when my breasts made their appearance on my chest. The fourth grade was a scary time for the entry into womanhood to commence. However, I reveled in the idea of being one of the only girls with such medallions of maturity. I suppose it was that very reason that I began to enjoy the extra attention boys were giving me. It seemed like such an easy way to get them to follow me around and do whatever I wanted them to. It was during this time that I began the long road of learning how to manipulate the opposite sex with my femininity. Though I felt like it was a sign of being in control, in truth, it served as the opposite. The attention I garnered over my young breasts, and later the rest of my body, became a self-induced prison.

Fast forward four years. All the other girls had breasts now, too. Somehow mine had managed to stay the size they became from the get-go, and everyone else's were much bigger. The once-treasured rarity of my breasts was a distant memory. It was apparent that most males I was surrounded by were fascinated with the size of boobs and so I developed a feverish jealousy over the girls with the much larger ones. To compete with the naturally larger breasts, I began to wear bras that enhanced the size of my chest. They weren't overly-pushup, but they were enough that it may have been a shock to someone who was used to seeing me with clothes on, to experience my true nakedness for the first time.

Around this same time, my then-boyfriend and I were on a mission to explore sexual adventures. I remember feeling nervous. What if he didn't like my tiny ladies once he saw them bare? What if the fantasy of what they would be was more exciting than the actuality of them?

Would he make fun of me? Would he still want to be with me? Thankfully, everything went off without a hitch and I found my boobs to be a useful tool yet again. He would do anything I wanted as long as he could see me naked. Oh, hallelujah! The skies opened up and the heavens poured down rays of sunshine over my insecurities. It seemed the itty-bitties weren't so bad after all.

Word spreads quickly around a high school. Sex is a powerful thing in the teenage world. As I remember it, once the boys knew I was keen on the sex thing, they all wanted a piece of me. Yes. Exactly. One piece of me. That physical rapture that can only be conjured by a female's soft body against theirs. At the time, it was extremely appealing to me to be held in regard for the pleasure my body offered. There wasn't any feminist raging in my head about me being worth more than that. It was the most exciting tool in my tool belt. Guys would literally follow me around like little puppies do. Honestly, that sort of validation was addicting to me.

That addiction continued to grow. But where did it come from? What was I truly seeking by gaining validation from the opposite sex? Looking back, what I thought I wanted was attention. Somehow I had created a reality where attention equaled love. It equaled acceptance. What I know now is deep down, I was hoping to find someone who would tell me I was good enough. It never felt like I amounted to much, from my own perspective. I always felt like I was lacking in intelligence, beauty, and every other quality a woman is supposed to have to be considered desirable. But why? Why did I feel so useless?

As many women can attest to, I had a difficult relationship with my father. His high expectations of me and hopes for me left me feeling incomplete. I was an adventurous tomboy, but he wanted a princess who sat still with a smile on her face. I was good, but not quite good enough. I was smart, but I could be smarter. I was pretty, but I wasn't as skinny as he hoped I would be. And he reminded me of these things regularly. The worst blow to my self-esteem was his desire for me to be an athlete. I was the farthest thing from it. My heart rejoiced when I participated in choir and art. I was aflame as a poet and a writer. Those were my natural gifts and they fulfilled me in ways nothing else could. I didn't understand or enjoy sports but to him, those were just excuses. My lack of desire to participate in sports was unacceptable to him. So, I did what any child desiring their parent's validation would have done; I sucked it up and I played. It wasn't my niche. I didn't excel. Not surprisingly, that only furthered his frustrations with me. He wanted me to be all the things I wasn't and he couldn't have cared less about the things I was good at.

Some part of me has been struggling since then to overcome that constant state of disappointment he drilled into me over and over again as a child. Why was I so unlovable to him? How could he only muster up the attention I craved when I was doing things that pleased him? Wasn't being his daughter enough? Unconsciously I decided if he wasn't proud of me, I never could be either. And because he was unwilling to give me the love and appreciation I so desired, I sought it from every other man I came in contact with. Whether he meant to or not, my father instilled the idea in me that it was my job to make him happy. Along with that came the conclusion that I was responsible for making every man I engaged with happy, as well.

My body became a useful instrument in this game I had created. There's nothing that makes a man happy quite like a naked woman who wishes to please him. This garnered me control in my relationships with men. They all loved my body, even when I didn't. I didn't see my body as beautiful or valuable, I saw it as collateral. So I used it to trade sexual pleasure in return for love. Or at least, that was what I thought I was doing. It turns out when you manipulate people, in any way, your plans don't quite turn out like you think they will. Even though men love to be pleased, they don't appreciate the energy that surrounds being used. When I found that I wasn't receiving fulfillment, no matter how much I tried to trick the love out of them, I ran. My demand for the continual replenishment of the thing I called love, kept me moving from man to man. Each man I took advantage of ended up as an afterthought as I moved on to the next. I needed to keep my deep abyss from getting deeper. I needed to fill the void. More sex, more attention. I repeated this cycle over and over again with many different people.

I pulled resentment and anger out of the men I was using, and my denial of these patterns grew as I tried harder to extinguish the burning ache within myself of it never being right, never being enough. It was as if I was punishing them in the way my father has punished me for years. I gained their trust, built them up, and left them guessing what they could have done to love me better. Then I moved on and they were stuck with feeling the emptiness and the loneliness of not being able to please me, the same way my father did to me. Because they became his replacement in my search for love, they also suffered the wrath I felt toward him. They endured the treatment I wanted to inflict upon him in my vengeance. I've left a trail of broken hearts in my wake, simply because I was trying to fill a void that wasn't able to be filled by sex and twisted versions of love. The game I created to get the love I wasn't willing to give myself ended up returning me shame and anger. The worst part was, I never actually got the love I was seeking to begin with.

At the time when I was lost within my self-serving madness, I couldn't see what I was doing. I couldn't face the truth of the cycles I was recreating again and again, or the damage it was creating. Today, I see the intricate webs I weaved. I see how my part in it was cruel and unfair. Instead of making myself wrong for it, however, I am able to change those behaviors that were so deeply entrenched in me. I am able to make thoughtful choices. I no longer abuse my body by trading it for false hope or to con men into games no one can win. Giving up the constraints of a bra is just one of the many I ways I choose to be kind to my sweet body. It still loves attention and it loves to be kissed, embraced, and pleased. However, I don't accept those gifts with conditions attached anymore. I have a loving husband who walks by my side as I make my way through uncovering and changing my bygone behaviors. And as I continue to reveal the truth within the lies I've told myself for so long, I am willing to do whatever it takes to be honest with myself and place my needs first in a way that isn't harmful to others.

As I practice new patterns of behavior, I find my body is responding with great joy and appreciation. When I am in the space of being willing to receive genuine contributions of love, I am fulfilled. I have become much more receptive to being honored and loved by others, but more importantly, I have found that I must be willing to do that for myself. Seeking beyond my own body for the love I deserve no longer serves me, when all I have to do is look within to find all that I desire. To say it has been challenging would be an understatement, but the value I find in me, as I truly be, is worth every minute of the process. Today I ask questions when I begin to feel old habits creeping over me. Am I being kind to myself? What does my body require? If I have feelings that seem unfamiliar or uncomfortable, I ask if they are even mine to begin with. When they are not, I return them to sender with consciousness, so the pattern can stop for them, too. Nurturing my body is not only valuable to me, it creates an energy of peace and strength for everyone that comes in contact with me. I am so grateful for all the pieces to my puzzle that have gotten me here, in this place of continuous consciousness.

Elisabeth Schweiger

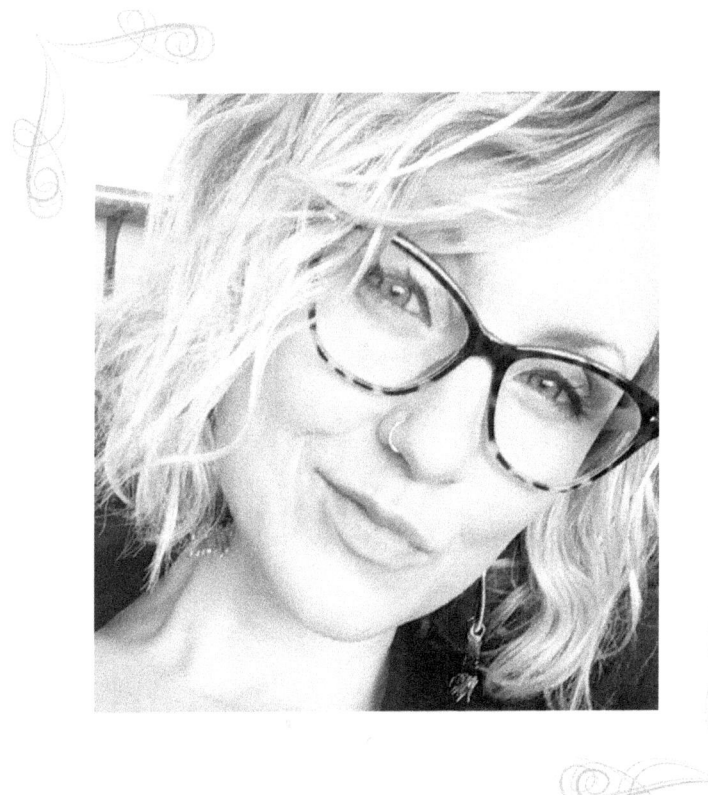

Elisabeth Schweiger *is a seasoned creator of magic! She is a Transformation Guide that specializes in energy healing, coaching, and organizing. When she isn't engaged in working with others, you can find her hiking, cooking, writing, or traveling. She resides in Madison, WI with her husband and two children.*

CHAPTER 7
TURN IT UP! TURN IT UP!

Kim Coleman

Do you know what I mean when I say, even though I am a beautiful lady inside and out, at one time for a loooooong time, for many years, I was really masculine? Yup! I spent a lot of years in my masculine energy showing my masculine side to the world.

I swore like a truck driver, behaved somewhat tomboyish and did my best to be like 'one of the boys'. Tough, hard, not weak like what was perceived in this reality that girls were. I never wore a dress or anything pink or lacy or pretty. I avoided looking or being feminine to the max (which to some, shone through regardless of my efforts to hide it even though I never gave myself permission to be it). My winter attire was a black leather jacket with my now ex-husband's plaid hunting jacket over it to keep me warm. I could spit really far, whistle with my fingers in my mouth really loud and shoot a hand gun or rifle with spot on accuracy. I was proving to myself and others that I was not weak just because I was a girl and had boobs. Oh wait, I even adorned a small

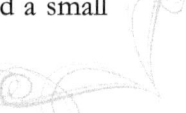

jackknife on my black leather belt in a black leather case for a few years. Oh yeah baby, I was a force NOT to be reckoned with. At least that was what I wanted everyone to believe. It was how I protected myself.

Now here is what is fun for me now. When I share that with folks who never knew me back then and are new in my life since those days, they are in 'full out full on' disbelief that someone as feminine, sensual and 'girly' as me could ever possibly be masculine. Yum! I love that response! It is then the norm that they giggle as they share that crazy idea with others, that I was once very masculine. Back at the time, had you said I was more masculine than feminine, I am not sure I would have known what you meant! Cause wait a minute. I have a pretty face, long beautiful hair, a nicely shaped petite body that I still keep fit and I was born with a vagina and eventually grew small breasts. So how could I be anything other than female. Ahhhh... see? That is the difference. Yes, I was born with a female body, however I was not feminine at all... those may have been fighting words, well, verbally anyway.

I think it must have been when I was in my late late 30s that something shifted. Some kinda magic or something happened. And wow, did something inside stir or what? Oh yeah, when the feminine fire ignites it is life changing. Of course, we are always in choice. For me, it was an intensity that was impossible to ignore with a potency that was beyond yummy! And I chose to turn it up!

And guess what that looked like? OMG not only did everything in my life change, even my body changed. My body became more feminine looking. I even began to grow fuller boobs. My face became softer looking. My body looked and moved completely different, so much so I signed up for and loved bellydancing and to my surprise, I was really really good at moving my body in such feminine sensual ways.

My relationships changed as I became such a different person, many ended and others began. Oh, even my clothing changed and I started wearing pink! My interests changed completely. My spidey senses (defined as a sixth sense of awareness derived from the superhero Spiderman) senses, my healing capacities, my awareness, my psychic knowings became not only the norm, they became my life and living.

My connection to the Universe, to nature, to the earth and to myself expanded beyond anything I ever thought possible. I began to radiate from the inside out and I began to turn even more heads. I got noticed by men, by women, by children. I got seen in a way I had never really acknowledged or noticed before. All of a sudden, I had a presence that became like a tsunami, a tsunami of feminine potency, sensuality and consciousness and more, which is undefinable even to me. I was purring inside and out, oozing and allowing myself and my body to be me! Regardless of how it was defined by this reality or how I was judged by others.

Oh yes! THAT! What if we all, men and women, penis people and vagina people, just simply allowed ourselves to show up without defining whether we are being masculine or feminine? How would we be different without all those definitions?

Somewhere along the line early on as a child, I had learned and concluded that to be feminine, would mean to be weak, maybe too emotional, and to be really girly would mean to be like the dumb blonde, not so smart. Oh wait. Wait. Also there is the one where if I am sensual and flirty, I am a slut or a whore. OUCHIE MAMA! No wonder so many women AND men have simply not allowed their softer feminine and sensual essence to show up. Men are often judged as gay if they show up that way in their creative side or their flamboyance fun and playful side. And frig, remember 'big boys don't cry'! I remember a song when I was young that the chorus line was Big Girls Don't Cry! I had three older sisters and I couldn't wait to be older like them and grown up, so if BIG girls don't cry then I was determined to NOT allow myself to cry either, no matter what. So I toughened up and sucked it up. Expressing our emotions that way was what? YUP! Considered a trait that girls expressed, big girls don't cry and men are wimps if they do. Wowsers, no wonder we have so many stressed out people with trigger points galore just waiting for someone to push that button and bam, explode all over the place. Messy shit right there folks!

Well guess what? This tsunami of feminine essence is here and YOU are soaking in it right now. Haha! Where are you NOT allowing yourself to receive that and to be all of that? This planet has been functioning from more of the so called masculine traits for a looong looooong time and now the feminine is sweeping the planet and everything on it. For both males and females. Maybe it IS time for us to just simply allow ourselves to be all that we be, regardless of what it looks like to others. Where are you sooooo hard-wired to what is considered masculine and what is considered feminine? What if you just allowed yourself to friggin' BE? Without all the definitions, limitations and boxes? Oh la la! Yes! More of that please!

Does consciousness have a gender? Does Infinite Being have a gender? True that if I have a vagina and breasts I definitely have a female body. How much fun can I have expressing all of me, ALL OF WHO I BE, in THIS yummy body? How much fun can YOU have being and showing up the same in your yummy body whether it has a penis or a vagina?

So here is what is super cool. Being that I am in allowance of my feminine side AND I am aware of my masculine side, I get to allow both and be both. I get to turn up either. It is not even something I actually have to do. It is simply who I be. I dare you, the reader. Play with this. If you notice yourself showing up and being what you may consider too feminine, or what is considered masculine, TURN IT UP! Just for fun, just for the experience without judging it or making it wrong. Just allow it and ask it to turn up even more and it will! At times I have entered a room and I am aware that others are not sure how to receive me, or if they even want to. I am also aware that by default in the past, I would begin to turn myself down a bit or a lot just to be able match where they were at in order to fit in or to be received by others. Now, I choose to turn it up and be the invitation for others to do the same, it's just a choice.

"Sometimes I've been to a party where no one spoke to me for a whole evening. The men, frightened by their wives or sweeties, would give me a wide berth. And the ladies would gang up in a corner to discuss my dangerous character."

~ Marilyn Monroe

Personally when I notice this type of reaction towards me, I become the invitation for them to shine even brighter, for them to come out of their box of feminine sensuality and potency, as I turn mine up and approach the ladies, including them even when they are not including me. And yes, in the beginning it was uncomfortable as I was aware of the refined judgements. Are you willing to be uncomfortable and go beyond even that? Are you willing to allow others to be uncomfortable around you if that is what they are choosing? Can you be you even then? Or do you turn you down? What if you became more aware of when it is a contribution to you to turn it up, and what if you became more aware of when it is a contribution to turn it down. It's just a choice. However, it becomes a choice, based on awareness, instead of autopilot or default.

"Life shrinks or expands in proportion to one's courage." ~Anais Nin

As you allow yourself to receive and be both the masculine and the feminine, you have so much more available to you. So much more ease, so much more fluidity in your body, so much more awareness, more and more of your capacities and magic can show up. When I am out in the world, if I find myself in a place that appears to be a bit sketchy, I turn up my awareness, my intuition, my spidey senses – all considered more of the feminine side of the brain. I also turn up my masculine side. I am in total awareness however am also without a doubt, ready to be a warrior if need be. I am not the feminine woman who is a potential victim who cannot defend myself. That is NOT the energy I am being or projecting in those moments. I am being all of me and with that, ALL of my capacities are available. I have the 'I see you, I am aware of you, mess with me and I will kill you' energy! And yes, I have been in THOSE situations more than once or twice or three times. Each time, I manipulated the entire situation to be exactly what was required by being aware of what that would take, what energy, what space, what consciousness me and my body could be to get out alive. Literally!

Yet wait a minute here. IF I have defined what is masculine and what is feminine and only allow in and be what this reality's version of that is, am I cutting off a part of what is actually available? BAM! Yes that! I would do that for what reason? If I can allow and be both and more and choose to turn it up, holy moly. I can use it to create and to generate and to contribute in so many more ways than I ever thought possible!

Are you willing to use your feminine sensual yumminess to create change on this planet? So many women are not, perhaps because of all of the pre-conceived notions of what being a girl or a lady means. It came as a gift as well as a curse for many women as we agreed and aligned with those judgements or notions.

Question: IF we all, men and women, allow more of the feminine essence that is begging us to receive it, how do you think that might impact the planet?

We call the planet 'mother earth'. Ok, so let's play with that for a minute. The feminine on this planet has been judged and shut down for a loooong time, in other words we have shut it out for a gawdzillion reasons. Does the earth have more life force now or less? What is happening to the earth herself as we ourselves have shut down, resisted and stopped the feminine that is within us and all things? Crazy idea? Interesting, as we receive and allow more of the feminine energy does that in turn, avail more of it for the earth to enjoy and feed on as well for her healing, her harmony and her nurturing? Could we possibly be the 'jumper cables and catalysts for that'?

And look at the sun! The majority of people on this planet have been functioning more from what we call the masculine. The sun in many cultures is considered male while the earth is considered female. How has all of this masculine energy that has been dominant on the planet influenced the sun? Has it come out of what we would call harmony? Has it become so strong and intense that it is actually considered dangerous? With all of the masculine energy being predominant on the planet, have we somehow energetically overcharged the sun? Is it out of balance? Now that is a lot to take in!

Could that be why there is this tsunami of feminine essence soaking the planet now? Could that be why more and more people are becoming what is considered intuitive, becoming more aware and psychic, more compassionate, people looking for 'spirituality and consciousness', more healing arts and modalities being created and received, more more more of all of those traits that are considered of the feminine? What if the earth requires it? Requires US to allow the feminine energy so that it can also nurture her and bring both her and the sun back to harmony? Many of us have been choosing to heal the earth, to connect with her and to create something different for a long time. Science tells us that everything is energy first. What if in allowing and receiving this feminine energy for ourselves, it actually contributes to and heals the earth and the sun bringing everything back to balance and harmony, including ourselves?

TURN IT UP PEOPLE! TURN IT UP!!

Don't you love how the little boys and girls are showing up now? The girls are really embracing their feminine side with all this princess stuff and what sometimes appears over the top girly stuff. What do they know? I love how even the little boys are desiring to wear pretty dresses too! What do they know? Are they both, the girls and the boys, more willing to be who they be, regardless of what body they are in? Have they come here to show us something totally different? Are they creating harmony and healing the planet as well as all of the beings on it, just by being them? Are you willing to allow that and whatever the expression of that looks like? How many parents, grandparents and others won't allow the boys to cry, to play with dolls or dress up 'like a girl' thereby defining, judging and limiting what is actually possible so that their kids fit in? Really? Do we want this reality to stay the same or would it be fun to enjoy more beauty, more compassion, more healing, more creativity, more awareness and all of the other capacities considered to be of the feminine? Einstein's definition of insanity is 'doing the same thing over and over again and expecting different results'.

OHHHHH! And have you noticed how many men are also incredibly intuitive, psychic, aware, choosing more consciousness, working with energy and the healing arts? These were all considered feminine traits in the past. YIPPEE! IN THE PAST! No longer defined by what this reality considers male or female. Let's just stop all that noise. Be an infinite being with a male or female body and not limited by its definition.

So whether you have boobies or not, whether you have a penis or not, this feminine energy is here and you are soaking in it. Yes I am an infinite being with a female body that I appreciate and actually really enjoy! My body and I know how to express and be sensuality, and it is super fun and yummy. And yes I can also allow what used to be considered my masculine ways to show up with ease as well. I get to allow it all, play with it all, be it all without defining it or limiting me! These are interesting times indeed and you being aware of when you are NOT allowing yourself to show up, truly is what this world requires. It is what we have been asking for and it is what creates something totally different!

I now absolutely love being a feminine lady. It is interesting to me how many women have soooo lost touch with the feminine and they ask me to give them a few suggestions on what they can do to allow it more. Keeping it short and sweet, I wondered what might be a couple of suggestions I can offer you here for both men and women.

- Is your home yummy? Do you have an aesthetically pleasing space? This is a nice place to start and it does not have to cost a lot of money. I love it when I find something that brings on that Mona Lisa smile to my lips and to my being. For me I usually have fresh flowers somewhere in my home that I can totally delight in their beauty. I recently purchased a canvas painting for about $29. The painting is an incredibly sensual woman, and every time I walk past her, I get that yumminess in my own body. Oh and I love my bronze statue of the goddess Venus, the goddess of love and beauty. One piece at a time I am creating a computer working space that feels sensually beautiful and alive to me. I get to luxuriate in each piece as I bring it home and place it. My next adventure is to create my healing room to be a classy exquisite space that oozes warmth and sensuality. Remember the inside of the genie bottle where Jeannie from 'I Dream of Jeannie' used to go? OMG that!

- Another 'thing' I really enjoy, is moving my body. I actually love watching myself as I do it! Now hang on there. There is a way that I do this. I put on my music that I like to dance to, which for me is usually pop music. I dim the lights way down low and I start to dance to whatever song is on the radio if I like it. I make my way over to the large window and that is how I watch myself. It is amazing how my reflection in the window with the lights down low makes my body look! I really enjoy watching my reflection, my moves and my body. Ha! Bodies love to move and they love to be appreciated. When you appreciate your body, your body will respond and appreciate you back. This is a fun and easy way for me to do that, which yes took time in the beginning and maybe even a glass of wine! Sometimes my clothes come off, sometimes they do not!

- Oh la la! Now when I apply lotion on my body, I do it with love and appreciation. I slow down, I don't do it from the place of 'gotta get 'er done', I use a sacred gentle touch. I use lotion that is natural and organic and feels really good on my skin. It is a contribution to my skin and to my body and I love it. I look in the mirror while I am loving my belly with the lotion. My belly carried my babies, it is sacred and I touch it as that. Nearly every inch of me (no not there, there is a different lotion for there) receives this lotion. Oh, now here it comes. As I am applying the lotion to my breasts, I allow myself to enjoy the sensuality of touch. I am not prodding or digging fearfully looking for lumps. I am more gifting myself with a goddess massage. I am doing this every day. IF there was something there that shows up different, I will notice it from this way of being with my body.

There are so many more ways I could share with you about how to really invite and allow the feminine, that in the past, has been shut down.

- I begin my morning with a cup of coffee in a mug that is not just any ol' mug. My mug is beautiful to me, it is something I look forward to being with as I awaken, it brings a smile on my lips as I sip from it, hold it and glance at it.

- I also invite you to explore each and every inch of your body.

- Start to become aware of which fabrics feel delicious on your skin instead of purchasing clothes just because they are cheap. Yes, your body and being will honor you all day and all night in your sweat pants, pajamass, work clothes or jeans if the fabric is a 'yes' to your body. They are each a contribution when they feel amazing!

- How can you even make eating an experience? Slow down and delight in your food, savouring every bite as if you are making love to it.

- Choose sheets, pillows and bedding that caress and nurture your body as you slumber. Even the thought of going to bed can FEEL GOOD and SEDUCTIVE!!

These are just some offerings, pick something and just start, even if it is just one thing. Engage and invite all of your senses that are available to you and your body from everything that this jewel of a planet has to contribute, and in that, you are contributing to it as well. Surround yourself with and actually notice and receive the beauty that is everywhere. BE THAT! That *IS* sensuality 101.

Now I double dare you to turn it up, turn yourself on to life and be willing to be way, way, way too much for this reality! If you are wondering where is the love and beauty on this planet and 'wish' it would change, then stop doing the same old thing expecting something different to show up! I triple dare ya!

Oh and along the way if you notice you are out of your comfort zone, CONGRATULATIONS!!! Being willing to be uncomfortable IS creating something totally different! Thank you for yummin' it!

> *"And the day came when the risk to remain tight in a bud was more painful than the risk it took to blossom"* ~Anais Nin

Kim Coleman
Brilliant · Bold · Sassy · Classy · Exotic · Enchantress ·
Foodie · Wine Lover · Mother · Grandmother

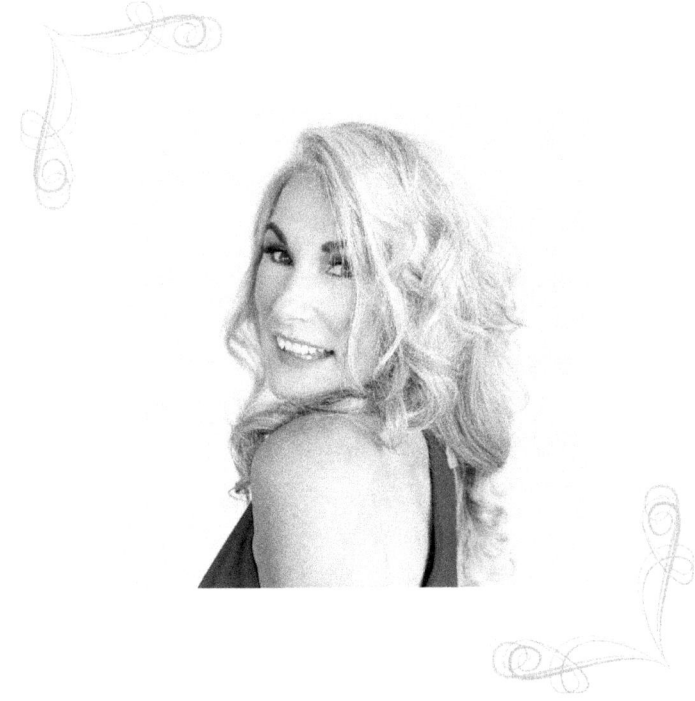

It is always been Kim's giggle and pleasure to spread gaggles of seeds of consciousness to those who are asking for it and choose it. For her that is her deal, it is beyond what Kim does, it is who she BE and how she shows up! Inviting women to be and allow their feminine sensual self is super fun whether on her table, in a class or a private session. Every cell in your body will wake up and you become more alive.

Her own personal life experiences enables her to be the space of allowance with just about anything. Kim has been facilitating classes in awareness, consciousness, energy healing and body processes since the early 90's with a list as long as yer arm. In 2004 she added Life Coach training with Coaches Training Institute (CTI) to her magic bag as well as Access Consciousness in 2011. Kim truly does create her life (since before she was born) as her unique expression of 'what else is possible' blended with her timeless and infinite expansion. She continues to boldly speak and share on numerous telesummits, radio shows and interviews as well as creating her own online teleseminars that go beyond the ordinary and what everyone else is offering.

What makes her unique is her clear and fun delivery of some of the most 'out there' information available today in the subject of consciousness. Her energy and her laughter is contagious and regardless of where she goes, she fills the room with her larger than large beyond energy. When working with clients, classes or during live calls she has this potent capacity to 'nail it', whatever the 'it' is in a style that will not only make you laugh, 'it' changes. One of the biggest comments that she hears is how folks never knew how easy, fast and gratifying it could be to be with some of their more difficult situations from the past to the present to create something totally different now and in their future.

Perceiving and knowing more, being and receiving more, showing up authentic and being different in the world has pretty much always been her way of, well, simply put… Kim… being Kim. And that is what is deliciously true for her! Being way too much for this reality and not fitting in are simply her norm. Are you ready for something totally different?

"Life isn't about going back to how things were when they were great, it is about creating forward motion from where we be in this moment!"

CHAPTER 8
A MODEL WEARS HER BREASTS WILD

Jennilynne Coley

*L*ights, camera, action! Chest out, chin down, smile with your eyes, shoulders back... those were some of the words I remember hearing on some of the film sets I've been on as an extra and on the photo shoots I modeled in. Everything had to be perfect and everything had to be just right. It was not okay to be too much... and it was certainly not okay to be not enough. I had to be PERFECT! What is perfect anyway? And does it even truly exist?

I remember watching everything I ate, working out constantly, having to keep my skin perfect... wrinkle free and blemish free, plus wear lots of makeup, and always stay on top of fashion trends. My ideal measurements were 34-24-34; a perfect size 3-4; a size 6 was really pushing it for any sort of dream of high-fashion modeling! While some of it was fun, a lot of it was stressful and I can only imagine how much I was torturing my body with all of that judgment, especially when my body tends to form muscles naturally, and muscles are the last thing that were socially acceptable for any respectable model.

Despite the fact that I was tall, slender, and gorgeous – everything a model was supposed to be – it was not sexy or OK to have muscles. So, I had to do pilates, yoga and lots of cardio, but weights were absolutely forbidden. I struggled to find the right personal trainer. I felt depressed a lot. But I desperately wanted to belong somewhere and since the modeling world was where I decided I belonged, I kept going and trying.

I was featured in a fashion segment on KUSI in San Diego with a designer named Leonard Simpson for a while, and I was in numerous photo shoots and other shows in Denver, San Diego and Los Angeles. Some of it was exciting and I felt like I accomplished something, and some of it was pure torture, waiting around for hours on end for things to begin, having to be happy, sad, excited, and many other emotions literally on command. What made it even more of a struggle was that I resented my beauty while at the same time forcing myself to embrace it…talk about a constant state of confusion. My last gig was posing for the cover of 303 Magazine in 2009. I was pregnant with my youngest child, although nobody knew it at the time, except the people I wanted to know. And I am often asked when am I going to start again, especially in a market like Colorado where you could literally model until you're 90 if you wanted to… it is the exact opposite of crazy, extreme markets like LA or New York. However, I truly have no desire to do so at this point. There's just something about asking to be judged that's not appealing to me at this point in time.

Right now I'm a size 8, and that could be considered plus size in some arenas, which means I'm essentially too fat for runway modeling and not big enough to be a plus size model… and I remember as a kid being too tall for children's clothing, but not tall enough for pre-teen clothing or modeling… too much and not enough simultaneously seems to have been the reoccurring theme… and my breasts have not been excluded. For the most part, they've always felt too small, except for when my dad told me they were too big because he likes small breasts… how's that for a total mind fuck? Especially from someone who's been oversexualizing you since you were a child. I remember him returning home from one of his six-month Navy deployments and the gift he brought home to his sweet, seven-year old child…a bright red Brazilian Bikini. As if society's conflicting messages were not enough, I was getting plenty of confusing ones right at home. And of course, I had no breasts at the time to fill that bikini out. I remember my mom always having larger breasts and really wishing I could grow up and have my own just like that. I would later find out that was very wishful thinking.

I was not an early bloomer by any means. I remember wanting my breasts to start developing and getting bigger when I was in the latter part of elementary school around fifth and sixth grade. With all the images and pressures we have as young women about our bodies and being desirable, this was something that was so important to me. In middle school, I was in a B-cup, and I still didn't feel like it was enough, despite all the modeling and what I now recognize as a killer metabolism. There was always this energy of never enough. But there were other areas where I was always considered too much. I was smart, so I was in gifted and talented classes in smaller select groups of students, most of which did not look like me. And I was constantly being told how my energy affected the entire room when I walked in so I needed to watch it and be aware of it. Yet, nobody ever told me what that meant or how to do it. So no matter what I did, I was wrong. I never felt pretty enough, lovable enough, developed enough, smart enough… even though school came very easy to me. And then I was constantly trying to figure out how to hide and be invisible so I wouldn't be too much and affect other people in the wrong way. What a confusing no-win level of insanity.

I experienced some sexual abuse at a very early age, and several times throughout my life after that. So, there was this ridiculous belief that I was only good for my body and my "beautiful face", and I hated that. I resisted it so much, not really understanding that it had managed to work its way into my subconscious as normal, as well as into the cellular memory of my body as familiar. And, no matter how much I ran, I could not escape from it. The abuse was attracted to me like a magnet, in my friendships, romantic relationships, work relationships. It was like I had a neon sign on my forehead that said, come here and use and abuse me any way you can. I'll go above and beyond to prove I'm loyal, lovable, trustworthy, more than just my body…so much so that I started ignoring it and separating from it.

However, there's life after creating all of that craziness and insanity. Yes, I did say that I created it, whether I consciously knew it or not. We create everything in our realities. So, once I was able to acknowledge that and stop buying into the addiction of a victim mentality, my journey to an actual communion with my body was able to begin. Now, it didn't happen overnight. But, it has been worth every minute, every ounce of effort, and every bit of ease I've experienced along the way. So, what does it take to actually move from victim and hating your body to loving it and being grateful for the gift of being alive?

Well, your journey may look a little different than mine. And, here's what I do know. Everything is energy. Remember chemistry class and the periodic table? Remember learning about atoms and molecules and cells in biology? What about friction, gravity, and the Law of Motion? Maybe you even made it to the study of quantum physics. Whatever you remember or don't remember, it's not as abstract as it seems. We breathe in oxygen everyday (two molecules of oxygen). We breathe out carbon dioxide (one carbon atom and two oxygen atoms bonded together). Our bodies are made up of over 80 percent water (two hydrogen atoms, one oxygen atom). We are energy. And our first language is energy. If you've ever heard a baby cry, and seen its parents respond, you've seen that without words that baby has managed to communicate with them, and the parents understood exactly what was going on by the vibration of the cry, hungry, tired, poopy diaper, colic, etc. And somewhere along the way as we learn words, we somehow seem to forget the subtle and simple ease that's available for us and our bodies when we receive the information of what we already are and know.

Think back to a time when you maybe made a decision and you had that feeling in your gut, or maybe a pit in your stomach, yet you did it anyway. That was the language of energy speaking to you. It's still available for you in any given moment. So, what about the energy and language of our breasts?

Our bodies are magical gifts that can heal themselves and tell us everything we need to know about what they desire or require. Bodies actually love to be touched. Did you know that an infant will die if it goes without human touch for too long? In reality, not much changes as an adult, although it looks very different. There are many benefits to paying attention to and gently caressing and massaging our own bodies, receiving and experiencing the gift of touch. More specifically, a breast massage has many benefits aside from pleasure, including anti-aging properties by releasing chemicals such as prolactin, oxytocin (decrease stress and depression), and estrogen, helping you look younger, and preventing sagging. Professor Tim Murrell, of the Department of Community Medicine, at the University of Adelaide says, "nipple stimulation encourages blood flow and promotes the production of a useful female hormone, which encourages cells to expel cancer-causing chemicals from breast ducts." With the incidences of breast cancer, I am all for doing what will decrease those chances.

There is a relationship with your body, especially your breasts, that can be very beneficial for every area of your life. So, one of the things that I recommend doing to enhance your relationship in this area is to really explore what you would like this relationship to look like. How would you treat your body if it was your child, your lover, parent, sibling or best friend? Would you feed it foods that actually make every cell of your body light up? Would you choose things that make your body joyful? Would you actually rest, when it's giving you signals that it would like to rest?

Take out a piece of paper right now and write down three things you are grateful for about your breasts and three things you are grateful for about your body in general. What could your life be like if you started to have more gratitude for the beautiful gift that your body is?

One of the things that I've started to do is to love all of my "imperfections". My stretch marks, cellulite, moles, oily skin in my t-zone, muscular build, and my not so perfectly straight teeth. These are all things that I obsessed over in the past. I even stopped making videos because my teeth used to be perfectly straight and I never had a lisp until a few years ago. I later discovered that I have a tongue thrust which has been slowly pushing my teeth forward and that created both the lisp and the imperfection in the straightness. And while I could go to speech therapy, and then get my teeth fixed, I consciously decided not to. I'm embracing it and loving me, just like I've learned to love my breasts just the way they are.

Right now my focus is on being HAPPY, exactly the way I am and raising my children. I'm enjoying my beautiful body and my breasts just the way they are. That's not to say that I wouldn't mind exercising for stress relief and my overall health, or even doing some toning here and there…my muscles naturally love being toned. However, the hardcore days are over. So what if I have a little cellulite. So what if I'm not a perfect size six or size four. So what if my breasts aren't the size of Mount Everest, and so what if sometimes my energy is! It's OK to be what people would call too much! It's OK to be what others may call not enough. It's perfectly OK to simply be ME! If I like me, the energetic signal I subconsciously give to others is exactly that…like me! Are you willing to like you? And I mean all of you, even the judgeable parts that you may want to change? Will you like you anyway? Especially your breasts…they are truly the first part of you to enter a room… wear them proudly!

I've developed the following acronym for my breasts to remind me when I have those down moments and I'm not thinking so clearly and judging them instead of being grateful for them?

B eautiful

R ound

E xtraordinary

A mazing

S ensual

T antilizing

What's funny is that I loved my breasts when I was pregnant, and especially when I was breastfeeding my babies afterwards. I was a DD for the first time in my life, lol! While it was fun to temporarily have my breasts that size, I knew my body could not support that long term. My back hurt sometimes because of it. Plus the pain of having too much milk in them (engorgement) was unbearable at times, and simply not worth the hassle. I also remember desiring a breast enlargement. However I have a slight problem that I honestly still haven't gotten over. I am terrified of being put under. I had a right pelvic hernia repair when I was a baby from deciding to throw a fit and pick up a vacuum cleaner. Silly girl, something must've gone terribly wrong because that fear of being put to sleep still hasn't left me. So, no matter how excited I was when the procedure came out when they could put the breast implants in through your belly button, it wasn't worth overcoming that fear. And now, I'm so glad I didn't. The idea and thought of some solution filled bag inside my body just absolutely makes me cringe. Not to mention my body absolutely despises foreign objects.

I've had my tongue, nose and belly button pierced, and they are all gone. Why? Because my body does not react well to foreign objects. They never quite healed up right, no matter how clean or dry I kept them. So, I stopped piercing my body, no matter how cute they looked and I stopped allowing any sort of "foreign objects" to enter my body. Thank you, body, I got the message loud and clear and I am so sorry I didn't ask you before I put gaping holes in you that later had to heal and close up. It always amazes me in life that people change one of two ways. Either slowly over time, or when something sudden or drastic enough occurs to almost force a change. It's the same way with our bodies, often times, but what if it truly doesn't have to be so. What if we could actually do something silly like ask it a question BEFORE we make a choice that might not work for our bodies? Try it, I dare you! And see what begins to show up!

So now I say no thank you to the stores who incorrectly size our bras, to give women some false sense of their breast size and make them shop more. I say no to the stores that incorrectly size women's clothing to make them feel smaller to improve their self-esteem and shop more. I say no to the lies about body image that are fabricated in our society today. At one point in time, it actually was attractive to be full figured and all the art of the times said so. So, who had it right, the past art or the modern-day magazines? And does it really matter? When do we as women stand up and decide what feels good and right for our own bodies, regardless of what society says? When do we ask our bodies what they'd like to eat, wear, sleep, go, etc? And when do we begin to drop the judgment and the lies and say yes to what lights us up, makes us come alive and just feels orgasmic? I wish I could say that I've come to these realizations overnight, but I have not. It has been a process over time that has involved a lot of things. One of which was walking away from judgment central, the modeling industry.

I would say that I have large nipples, great for breast feeding. And small to average sized breasts. They fit perfectly in my hands and I love that! I do not necessarily enjoy that when I begin losing weight, after my abdomen area starts to shrink, the fatty tissue in my breasts tends to be next. It's as if mother nature is playing a dirty joke. However, I've come to be at peace with how my body chooses to do things. Although, sometimes I really wish some of the extra cushion that loves to hide around my legs would gravitate towards my breasts, it truly is all good either way. My body is perfect for me. What if your body is also perfect for you? And what if you could always be willing to ask your body questions about what it desires and what it requires in any given moment?

For years, I hated wearing "regular" bras. I would only wear sports bars. For me, they feel more comfortable, less restrictive, and what I did not know at the time is that research also shows that they remain perkier when you ditch the underwire! Did you know that? And, I'm still willing to ask my body questions. So, I actually own both "regular" bras and sports bras. And depending on what I feel like wearing on a particular day, that's what I choose. I must admit that my favorite is no bra at all, so once I get home the bra comes off, no matter which one I wore that day. And, on occasion when I go out, I leave the bra at home. What if you no longer had to play by the "rules" that God knows who made up at some point in time? What feels good for you and your body? What if it's not about being or looking "sexy" as if that's some sort of badge of honor that you must always uphold.

Now, don't get me wrong, sometimes dressing and feeling sexy is AWESOME! I do notice that when I wear certain clothes or dress a certain way, I stand a little straighter, I feel a little happier and everything just seems to flow with more ease. And, I truly believe it's not because of the clothes. I believe it's an energy that starts within me and then the clothes I choose to wear match that energy and contribute to expanding it. So, what if we could all learn to listen to our bodies, remember our first language of energy and trust it and create every area of our lives from the possibility and magic of that creation?

My breasts love being touched. My nipples love being stimulated and pinched, even during sexual encounters. It sends a tingle down my spine and lots of orgasmic energy through my body. Sometimes, I even enjoy just holding my breasts in my hands in a totally non-sexual way. It's like giving them a hug and saying thank you for being a part of my body. God made them and gave them to me, so why not be grateful for them. For me, it's no different than caressing my arm, clasping my hands, twirling my hair or gently caressing my thigh. When did it become taboo or unacceptable to provide ourselves with the same amount of nurturing, caring, physical touch and attention as we would a newborn baby? What is it that your body truly enjoys? What is it that would actually work for you? How much freedom could you experience if you stopped judging you and just did what actually works for you?

My final words are six tips that can create you having greater ease in your relationship with your breast s and your body.

6 Tips for Having Ease With Your Body:

1. Eat the damn cake!
2. Create a life you love that's full of a lot of joy
3. Honor your body with the gift of touch (babies)
4. Speak your body's love language
5. Move, move, move – magic and energy that gets released and activated when you move
6. Stop torturing your body with chemicals and surgery

JENNILYNNE COLEY

Meet Jennifer Lynne Coley aka Jennilynne!

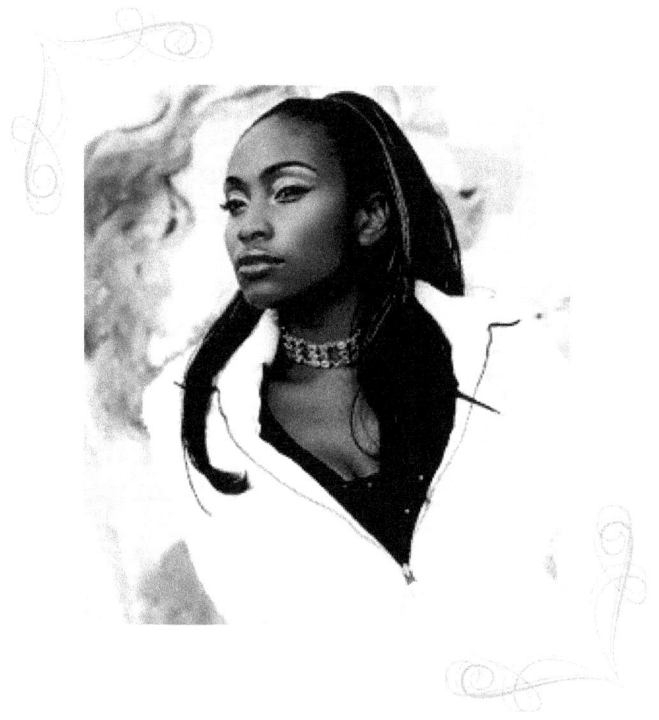

Jennilynne is lit up about education in all sorts of arenas, but not in the traditional sense. The root word of education, "educo", actually means "to draw out". And that fits beautifully with her take on education… the belief that we all have our answers inside of us… and that "point of view" has been precisely what led her to Access Consciousness®. She enjoys providing one-on-one sessions for her clients, as well as facilitating BARS® and Body Process classes. What better way to experience people activating more of them and drawing out their inner genius?!?!

Visit her personal website at http://www.accessyourgenius.com.

CHAPTER 9
VAGENI
Jeni Griffith Burgess

When I think about Breasts I think of Bodies and when I think of Bodies I think of Sex. When I think of my Sex I think of my Vagina. Yes, this chapter is the journey of courting and creating a relationship with my vagina. Most of my life it's been a painful relationship of disconnect, brokenness, and shame. This is my journey from shame, embarrassment, confusion and self-reproof to adoration, affection, and Love.

My story begins with innocent child-like curiosity. I was 5 years old and I remember sitting in the tub and feeling the hot water hit the lips of my vagina. A warm sensation filled my tummy and gave me a tingle. That was the first time I noticed my vagina respond with a sensation. This was very different from the sensations of my ears, nose or other body parts. I sat in the tub opening and closing my legs. It felt good and I really liked it. Similar to when my mom would tickle my back but very different. I just knew it felt good and was happy and proud of my 5-year-old discovery.

Something interesting occurred past the age of 7. My fun curiosity now became a secret curiosity. Cover up! "You are too old to be run-

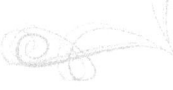

ning around like that!" It was never talked about or explained. It was now required that I keep my body covered and never let anyone see my naked body and especially not my vagina. Then the really bad news: My vagina shamefully referred to as my "privates" was now off limits. "Don't play with it. Don't touch it unless you need to wipe or wash it. And definitely, don't explore it and be curious about it. Leave it alone." I wanted to be curious about my vagina but it felt bad and wrong. Like a shameful secret. It was to be ignored and covered up. As time went on I would silently notice things about my vagina and make mental notes not to be shared with anyone.

I grew up in an extremely strict religious home. Every Sunday was church. Every night was family scripture study. Every morning was family prayer. Every Monday night was a gospel lesson. Every day I was supposed to have my own prayers and my own scripture study. It's an understatement to say I had weighty instructions on what was right and wrong, what was a sin and what was good. I was taught Sex was bad before marriage and good after marriage. Sex was supposed to be "sacred". I never knew what the hell that meant. I remember hearing the word masturbation and being taught it was a very bad, shameful and dirty thing. It was something that boys did and they should never do it. If they did do it, they would have to repent because it was a sin. At that point, I didn't know what masturbation was or how boys did it I just knew it was very bad.

My first information about sex and came from a planned conversation at 8 years old. My uneasy parents gave the "sex talk" out on the front steps of our house. I specifically remember the steps being very cold on my butt and vagina. And very hard! I was given the science version of the sex talk. The talk begins with the seed fertilizing the egg. Daddy had the seed and Mommy had the egg and that's how babies are made. My Mom's flustered end to the talk was "do you have any questions?" I sensed how uncomfortable she was and I responded with a quiet "no." I wanted to ask questions but it didn't feel safe. The awkward silence and unanswered questions left me confused and keeping my curiosity a secret.

I vaguely remember the maturation talk at school. My mental note was something about when hairs start growing on the top of your vagina you know your period is close. You better believe I was watching for that.

I had an older sister and I knew she had her period every month because she complained about it. My parents complained about her attitude. I knew my mom had a period, they both used pads and it wasn't pleasant.

A few years later the door to my secret curiosity was ever so slightly opened. I sat in a circle of 10-year-old girlfriends playing "truth" on the trampoline. One of the girls asked, "truth, how much hair do you have growing down there?" The first girl shyly said, "I have a little hair down there." The next girl boastfully said, "I have a lot of hair down there." We all gasped! You do? You have a lot. Wow, cool. There it was, A crack! A crack in the closet of my secret curiosity

I was 11 years old two months before my 12th birthday when I received the jolting shock of a reddish brown stain in my underwear. The self-discovery and surprise began a string of racing thoughts like a runaway balloon. What is that? Did I poop my pants? No that's not poop. It doesn't smell like poop. Is that blood? Is this my period? I wiped my vagina with toilet paper. This looks more like the color of blood. Yes, that's blood, ok yes this is my period. It's happening. What do I do?... I sat on the toilet looking at the earthquake in my underwear. This was a big moment. I didn't know how to process this. I wasn't even sure what all I was feeling. It was a big sensation that felt overwhelming. I was scared and feeling lonely with my vagina. With a blank stare, I went through the motions of changing my underwear and laying a pad down so I didn't get my clean underwear all yucky. I then told my older sister in a half excited way resembling bragging. I secretly hoped she would somehow know how to talk to me about it. Dismissively she said, "Oh, well, good for you, you should tell Mom." Telling my Mom was a like having a talk about the responsibility of cleaning the bathroom. She plainly asked, "You know where the pads are?" "Yeah," I said. "Alright," she said indifferently. "Be sure to clean out your underwear, so they don't stain." "I already did," I said. She responded with "you're all set then." No acknowledging or asking me how I felt about it. It was like learning where the toilet cleaner is stored. I felt alone. From her nonchalant response, I learned that this is another part of being a girl that should be ignored. I was to take care of it, clean it up and carry on.

In my mind, the words "clean it up" were burned into my memory and now my once fun tingling vagina is now a smelly dirty place that I needed to keep clean.

That memorable day began the belief that my vagina is to be kept clean and not cared for or discussed.

If every part of my vagina was bad and shameful I certainly wasn't going to tell anyone about the sexual abuse I endured. If I couldn't even ask a question and be curious. I didn't dare speak about it. The colossal amount of shame of my vagina branched throughout my body. To disconnect from the pain I disconnected from my body. I emotionally detached from my vagina and safely created a separation I could live with.

Around the age of 13, I learned about masturbation and how boys did it. I didn't know that girls could masturbate. I didn't even know what a clitoris was or that I had one. I knew I had a vagina to be kept in the dark covered and clean and untouched. I did leave it alone and never looked at it until I put in my first tampon.

Fast forward a few years and what was left of my secret curiosity became a secret pleasure. In my family, we prayed a lot. Every morning before school we kneeled in a group on the floor and someone prayed on behalf of everyone present. I had 8 siblings so it was a large group of bowed heads and folded arms. One morning as I kneeled on the floor I noticed when I rocked side to side it felt really good. Suddenly I was keenly aware of the stitching in the crotch of my 501 jeans. It rubbed against my vagina and a warm sensation filled my pelvic area. I stealthy looked up to see if anyone's eyes were open. The coast was clear all eyes were closed. Ever so casually I sat back on my knees and rocked side to side. As I rocked I was careful to keep my eyes open to watch for popping eyelids. Lost in sensation the prayer ended and I had no clue what had been said nor did I care. At this point, I had been educated enough to know that I would not share this new found secret pleasure. I was afraid if I said anything they would get mad and tell me to stop. In case I got caught and was questioned I needed a reason for why I was rocking. My brilliant response was I had to go to the bathroom and a love affair with my 501 jeans was born.

Middle School health class we were taught about sex. There were bursts of giggles and plenty of embarrassing blushing. The anatomy of both boy and girl genitalia was discussed with a side slow presentation. Sex was a penis going into a vagina. Ok, got it I remember thinking. After class, I had a few conversations with girlfriends, mostly about our fears of sex. There was a disconnect with my vagina she remained clean and ignored. Once I learned about kissing I abandoned my vagina entirely as kissing was way too fun.

My love and enjoyment of kissing continued as I grew into my teen years. Somewhere in the back of my mind I knew kissing led to sex, but that was for boys. At 17 I knew the only way my vagina related to sex was that was where a boy put his penis and that's how you got pregnant. My limited knowledge of sex and an overflowing abundance of shame had me disconnected from my vagina. Of course, I wouldn't have sex until I was married. That's what I was taught and that's what I thought would happen.

My first sexual experience started with lots of kissing and touching. I remember him taking off his pants and saying "I'm going in" everything in my head came to a screeching halt. It was like someone had pulled the emergency brake and my world toggled between slow motion, freeze frame and fast forward. I thought "you're going in where?!" "I'm going in," he said again. "Ooooh, he's going in my vagina… Okay, I thought this is happening" A whiplash of 90 seconds and it was literally over and then "I'm pulling out" he said. There was such a complete disconnection to my vagina I did not feel much of anything. Disillusioned I realized I just had sex and now we have to get married, so we did.

That marriage ended and another began. I did this several times over the years. In my world, I didn't know there was any another option to be with a man sexually. My marriages created more disconnect and disillusionment from my vagina.

At 18 I had my first child. With that came nurses and doctors all looking at my exposed vagina. I had to get the baby out quick so my vagina could be cleaned and covered.

At 21 my first orgasm was a happy accident. I was having sex with my husband and all of a sudden what seemed like out of the blue something happened. I was like what the hell was that? Holy crap that felt good. OMG... I think I just had an orgasm. A storm of fireworks and stars and explosions. Years of Storm chasing had paid off. Desperately yearning for my husband to make it happen again during sex without the know-how, patience timing or finesse. I began to feel shamefully broken and despondent about my vagina. Why wasn't it working again? His thirty-second attempts to make it happen left me convinced my parts didn't work in sex. I was broken and my vagina did not work. My secret curiosity encouraged me to figure out how to give myself an orgasm. It was always a sight unseen experience. This became a painful secret of shame I kept to myself for years.

My quiet disgraceful and hidden conflict went on for over 20 years. I was sure something was wrong down there and there was definitely something wrong with me. I had many moments of giving up. This is just the way I am. This is what is for me. I must be the only woman in the world who is broken.

At 41, divorced and no longer involved in the strict religious lifestyle of my past I began to explore my sex.

In that exploration, I hit another level of shame as I realized I didn't know my own vagina. I didn't have any connection to the anatomy of what specific spot could bring me pleasure if I could even remove the shame and guilt long enough to feel pleasure. The judgment began here with repeating thoughts of 'How could I not freakin know about my own vagina for God's sake I've had a vagina for over 40 years'.

When I looked down at my vagina I saw the top of it. When I looked at myself naked in front of the mirror I only saw the front of it. Where is my vagina? Men seem to have a different relationship with their penis. Most men seem to very proud of their penis. They find it at a young age when their hands start exploring and don't let it go. I mean it hangs out in front and they see everything that is happening to it. I had seen my vagina in the mirror, I watched as each of my kids were born, but I never really looked at it, explored it or felt anything kind towards it.

One day things started to shift when I met a partner who loved my vagina. He verbally expressed his adoration for the beautiful shape of my lips that magnificently formed a heart. He was transfixed by the gorgeous colors of pink and amber. He gently explored each delicate fold like opening an enchanting flower. The softness of his eloquent exploring and alluring play of my vaginal beauty set off a silent angst within me. What was he seeing? I have never seen what he was sharing with me and I desired to connect with my vagina in the way I was experiencing him cherishing her. I wanted to adore and love my vagina that way.

This inspired my journey of my own exploration of my vagina. The spark of curiosity was renewed and coursed through me. I got a hand mirror and spent time with my vagina. My first attempts were vulnerable and confronting. I desperately wanted to switch my thoughts and just love it and I didn't. I was angry at my vagina. I blamed her for being so attractive and beautiful. Being a girl and having a vagina is what attractive the abuse. I'm still angry at her. I'm not over it. My desire to release my shame and anger guided me to start a daily practice. A daily practice of looking in the mirror at my vagina and saying out loud and acknowledging what I am seeing. I recently bought a notebook to journal what I am noticing and discovering. I am putting my attention on caring about my vagina, not just taking care of her. I am gently beginning to see her with a new set of eyes. I am realizing she is communicating with me. As I sit in silence in front of the mirror. I am starting to feel the nudges of her communication to me. In my budding practice, I'm seeing more celebration of noticing and less anger. I'm being introduced to see the exquisite beauty my partner saw. I am practicing learning to listen and She is gradually teaching me. I've ignored my vagina for so long and disconnected from her that this is unhurried process and experience. I am learning from my own vagina. I am dispelling the lie that I am somehow broken. I'm beginning to see and experience a world of pleasure and joy I once thought impossible. I don't have to search for it or find it. It's here in plain sight. I never stopped to notice and explore what is right in front of me. Is it all better now? Is the judgment gone? No, but it's better. It keeps getting better as I take the time to be with her in a loving way. I am starting to reconnect to the joy I experienced in the bathtub many years ago.

My hope is that my story will inspire you to look your own relationship with your vagina. Do you have one? What is your current relationship? Is it a relationship of adoration or is it a situation of keeping things clean and hidden? What is the last conversation you had with your vagina? The truth is you have a relationship because you have a vagina. The choice is what kind of relationship would create the most happiness for you, your body, your vagina, and your partner.

JENI GRIFFITH BURGESS

Speaker, Author, Teacher, Body Mentor, Life Coach,
A lover, A mother, A grandmother. A woman of strength and power. Full of Desire, Joy and passion.
Exploding with purpose

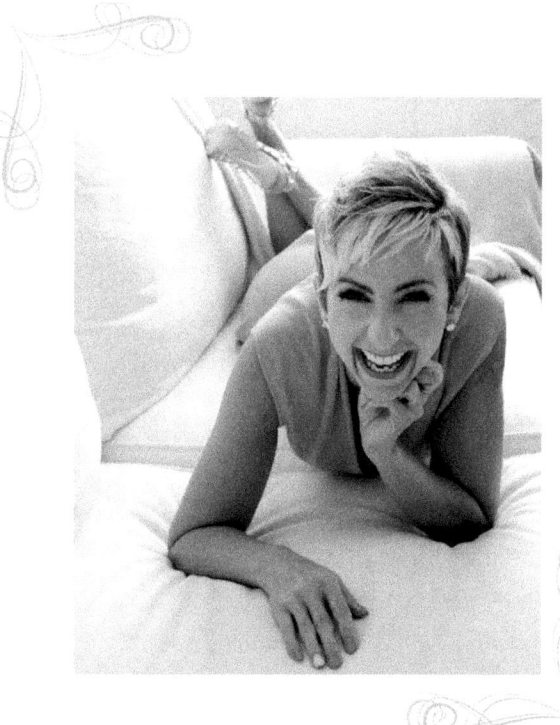

In all of the seasons and spots of my life, my greatest desire is happiness. I scaled through programs, institutions, organizations, authorities, belief systems and many realms of consciousness searching for permission to live by my choice. I guide clients to create a connection with their body and to navigate the sensations in their body. Navigate to freedom and choice. Being able to be present to and move through to the sensations in the Body is one of the greatest tools of awareness.

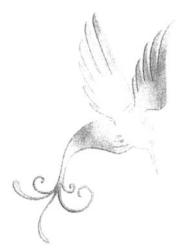

CHAPTER 10

I LOVE MY BREASTS!

Jennifer Lamkins

When I reached my late teens I was really beautiful. I had long svelte legs that my friends envied and muscles everywhere that showed off my curves. I seldom brag, yet I can honestly say from a vantage point 20 plus years in the future, that was true. I truly was sexy, beautiful, honest, vivacious, smart, funny, and imaginative, even if I didn't know it back then.

What I did know was that I was brave. I knew that if I could hold myself up that it would be less likely people would target me and possibly hurt me. So, I did confidently strut my stuff… on the outside. I liked to act tough and confident, but inside I never felt confident or very attractive. All of my flaws were very loud in the mirror when I looked at my reflection. Sadly, I was hyper focused on everything attached to my little bitty titties. I so desired to have big round breasts and I found it really embarrassing that when I would lie on my back, my overdeveloped rib cage was more pronounced; more perky than my boobs.

I was super aware as a young adult and VERY aware that most men found big breasts attractive. I had even more evidence of this at home

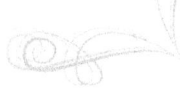

since my own mother was a beautiful blonde with large breasts who knew how to captivate and manipulate a room with her "personality".

When I was around 13, my mom and I would laugh as I pranced around the house with oranges she stuffed under my shirt just for fun. Like somehow we were doing a rain dance to get them to grow! It all seemed in good fun, but subconsciously left me in silent expectation of what was required and what I was not.

By age 16, I would lie in bed at night summoning my breasts to grow! If I only knew then that that judgment was probably a contributor to stalling any further development, I would have stuffed a sock in my mouth! If you would ask my parents, even today, they would excitedly tell you I was an obstinate child and I'm so very grateful for it! This streak of stubbornness, that grew stronger as I aged, assisted me in my motivation to push forward in the face of my need to be obediently people pleasing to everyone. As a child, I had such a need to gain other's approval I would oblige even when I knew that they were manipulating (or thinking not so nice things about) me. No one in my home knew anything about healthy boundaries, or self-care, so I initiated my own search for better role models. Like Wonder Woman! She was at least a brunette, like me; smart, like me; and had super powers, like me! (But… that will have to be a story for another time.) After watching Wonder Woman reruns in the late 70s and 80s, I decided that

> **Friends are like Boobs. Some are Small. Some are Large. Some are Real. Some are Fake.**

I desired to be strong, powerful and sexy just like her! I would still go in waves ranging from resentment to tolerance over being small chested. I thought for sure that when I was older I would get breast enhancements until I turned 16 and underwent oral surgery to correct my jaw misalignment. After that experience, which included 8 hours in surgery and over a year of recovery, I could easily talk myself out of any unnecessary surgery all the while judging myself insufficient in the endowment department.

My obsession with having larger breasts continued and so I tried water bras, pushup bras, and corsets. None made my breasts into D cups. I was still brunette and fairly flat chested. To make matters worse, I was born with a third nipple. Yes, you heard that right. A third nipple. The butt of so many jokes and the secret shame I carried for decades.

So much crazy around my body! But in the midst of all of that I won't lie to you and tell you that I didn't know somewhere inside that I was sexy! In fact, in my 20's I oozed sex appeal… which manifested itself in the very dark and dangerous variety mostly because of the hidden secret below my right A cup. Because of what I was hiding I was so fearful about being judged for my birth defect, the Scarlet "N" of shame, I chose to be very dominant in most areas of sex and the dance of captivating a man's attention. But, sadly, when things became more intimate, I cowered and became a flaccid body in the bedroom thinking, that was the price I had to pay to prove I was aware and embarrassed of my body. So alas, the biggest perpetrator of judgment was me. (This has only very recently shifted for me. Oh, the years I wasted not enjoying my body!)

Then one day in my early 20s, I was listening to a distant relative joking around about her body weight. She was saying that her excess weight had so many advantages! I perked up to hear how that was even possible to be stated in a group of my family, who were very disapproving about excess weight especially on the female body, so I was intrigued. She went on to say that she thanked her weight for her large beautiful breasts and why she always appeared so much younger than her true age because the extra weight hid her wrinkles. Everyone in the group laughed. I can't say for sure if she meant what she was saying, but I bought her logic and imbedded it into my system instantaneously!

Shortly after, I attracted into my life a man who enjoyed a more full-figure body and who encouraged me to gain weight. And, as I gained more weight, helped me receive my new look with ease. I had gained 30lbs in less than a year and my little A cup became a beautiful full B! I was ecstatic! Who cares if my hips had a bit more curves and my tummy more bulge! I had boobs! My bounty was then after affectionately referred to by me as *the ladies* I had been waiting for! I felt more confidence with my breasts there to accompany me wherever I roamed. In clothes; I looked good, I felt great, and when I entered a room, everyone knew I had arrived because my presence was energetically unmistakable. My best friend would even say that when I walked into a room I owned it! I will tell you secretly, that I didn't always feel the confidence that I portrayed. But, some days, whoa! I did feel good! In reverence to those days, I can replay it all comically in my head, like it was a scene from an old western… She shows up and her energy bursts open the saloon doors, she struts inside and sits down on a bar stool and looks down at her two smoking guns (as you see pistol smoke rising from both sides of my chest as if I was acting right beside Leslie Nielson). I felt sexy! I felt confident! I felt strong! I was Wonder Woman!

Then, later in my late 20s, my man and I parted ways after a tragedy in the family. We didn't manage our grief well and I became very depressed and put on another 30lbs. My breasts moved up from a B to a D cup which was the highlight of those events. Although I was happier than ever with my new chest and I proudly displayed my ladies in V-neck shirts, I really wasn't loving much more about my body. I was still desperate to find something to blame that I could "fix" that

The Perfect Man is like the Perfect Bra: Supportive, Sexy, and Washes Well

would help me feel better about myself. I had plenty; I was not in the best health for many reasons, one of which the doctor's reported that I couldn't conceive a child. This was such devastating news to me since all I really desired in the world was to be a mom. I was racking up more reasons that I wasn't good enough to be loved by me, much less anyone else faster than I could count them. My self-esteem plummeted and anywhere that I imbued the magic of Wonder Woman disappeared.

I was seriously in a state of constant panic as I searched for a way to alleviate the pain and rationalize how to make me good enough to love. I went on a drinking binge for about 4 years trying to numb myself, but knew that I was called to do more in this world. I didn't have enough tools to understand what that was completely, but I knew the drinking had to stop. When I wasn't numbing out with alcohol, I began again struggling with how to rationalize why I didn't love me; why I wasn't good enough for me or anyone else to love.

I wasn't ready to hear the truth yet, so I came to conclusion that my lack of confidence and self-love would be "fixed" if only I wasn't born with this third nipple.

I was also very lonely. I missed having a partner. I missed having a lover. AND I hated dating! I just wanted a romance novel worthy relationship! What I wouldn't give for a quick meet-cute and a short courtship! A man who would love me no-matter-what and I could finally stop judging myself for not being perfect, as long as I could be perfect for him. My fear of not being able to find someone to love me again with all my flaws, or worse yet, me not allowing someone to love me with all my flaws, was not good ingredients to meet the kind of man I truly wanted to attract as a life partner. So, I didn't date much and when I did it wasn't very successful. I attracted men who validated that I wasn't good enough to be loved. They definitely played their part in giving me opportunities to choose to be loving and kind to myself. I still hid in shame from my third nipple using it as the reason I was flawed and no one could treat me kind or love me the way I desperately craved to be loved.

In my early 30's I decided to brave the knife and have a simple surgery to remove my little companion. I thought that was going to be the magic wand to make me love my body and receive the sex, adoration and the acceptance that I desperately craved! I wish that I could tell you that the simple afternoon office visit changed my life and like magic everything was perfect, but that's not what occurred. After I removed my barely-there-nipple, I was only left with myself, which really, as it turns out, was the gift when I had been asking for all along. It brought with it some huge awareness's that I wasn't on a journey to fix my exterior, but instead needed to search inward to see all my broken pieces.

I read everything I could get my hands on about self-improvement. I did affirmations, and inner child work, and vision boards, and took tons of classes and achieved many certifications in energy healing for the next 15 years. In each of these experiences I became more aware that I am so much more of what I believe about me than what I saw in the mirror. Intellectually I completely got it. I stored all the information and was an amazing student, anxious to share all my knowledge with anyone who would listen.

I also lost the weight again, and some of my breast size, too. But I gained insight into what journey I needed to take to feel a true sense of sexy, confident and strong. I also got pregnant at 31, despite what the doctors said would be impossible. As I read more and more self-help books, I eventually met other people who worked with energy and healing that path led me to Access Consciousness® which really assisted to boost my inner confidence and remove layers of judgments. As I continue to travel this path, I also continue learning more about how to love myself at any body or breast size. I've had the joy of exploration on learning to love and receive more of me! (Which I have now accepted is a journey, not a destination!)

If Only Women Would Love their Breasts As Much as Men Do!

You see, it was never really about my breasts or any part of my body at all! It was always about how I felt about me inside and what I made important about who I was or wasn't. If I was taught more about how to love me then I may have received more of me sooner, but I won't blame my parents for not teaching me something they weren't taught. And, really, how lucky am I to be teaching my daughter a completely different way to be about her body!

Since I've taken such an interesting journey through how to enjoy the chaos of me as I weave through my stuff (to get to the good stuff!), I have learned a few things about not taking myself too seriously. If shit starts getting heavy in my world, I know I have some wounds to lick and more healing is available.

The best part about receiving, loving and healing more of me is that I get to receive more beauty, more awareness, and more… well, just about anything becomes available as I be more loving and gentle with me! Like the beautiful surprise bonuses I've been given, like the gift of also finding more people who desire to be more gentle and loving to me showing up in my life.

I still like Wonder Woman! But I no longer desire to be her. I am my own version of wonder. I have conquered more than my share of dangers and have cast away all sorts of villains. I am so grateful for each and every event that has occurred thus far. Each situation has given me an opportunity to choose me; love me; accept me; adore me; advocate for me; forgive me; praise me; and, receive me.

Since then I've been all sizes. I have had small breasts, medium breasts, large breasts, pregnant breasts, breastfeeding breasts and a little bit more on the sag breasts, and through all of the stages of *my ladies*, I love them! I love them so much for staying healthy! I love them for their bounce! I love them for their sensitivity and pleasure! I love them for being a part of me!

…And, you know what else…

They are always just perfect!

Jennifer Lamkins

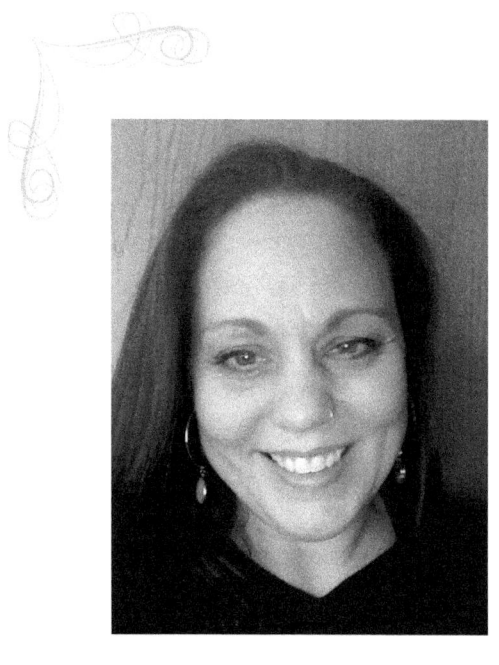

Jennifer *has lived mostly in the Fox Valley Area of Wisconsin for the last 25 years. Growing up as an intuitive psychic with a deep compassion for the wellness of others, she has devoted her life to learning natural health methods with a concentration on the power of energy frequencies. She has worked countless wellness events sharing her knowledge for the last 7 years.*

Currently, Jennifer owns and operates Transcendence Mind~Body~Spirit Ministries® in Appleton, WI. She is a practicing Empowerment Coach, Facilitator for Access Bars®, Hypnotherapist, Massage Therapist, Reiki Master, Ordained

Minister, Wellness Consultant for doTERRA© essential oils, Spiritual Body worker and Author. She has developed a technique called Multidimensional Therapies for Whole Body Health™.

A few components include integrating energy work, re-routing neuropathways by restructuring thoughts, and accessing trapped emotions to assist in their release using the tools of Access Consciousness® and many more modalities.

Jennifer loves teaching educational classes for individuals and groups. She teaches Access Bars Practitioner training, Reiki Level 1, 2, 3 and Master classes, Empowering Your Soul class and Intimately, Yours Truly class, to name a few.

CHAPTER 11
HAVING IT ALL
Brittany Rogozinski

*A*s I walk into my office with my full fat cappuccino and dark chocolate cherry bar, a memory washes over from my past of time where I would be having huge guilt about this, wondering how I could cut calories later and go to the gym, obsessing over my weight. Today I have no judgement, if I want to finish my drink I will finish it. If I want to have another later I will have another. I have decided I will not punish my body anymore, instead I will listen to it. I will make it happy. My childhood was a daze. I was in and out of hospitals gathering everyone's opinions and judgements, and making them my own. I had several surgeries where, in my interesting point of view, aided in locking these judgements into place. To top it off, my father, who is now a very kind and humorous gentleman, was just a young guy who let his emotions get the best of him. I was what in this reality would say "verbally and physically abused". I had always been told "You're too fat! Don't eat that! Exercise more!" for as long as I remember. It was these verbal processes that aided in my weight ballooning up to 300lbs. Not that there is anything wrong with that,

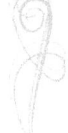

but it was not comfortable for me. My body was not happy. I was not listening to it, and on top of that I was taking on everyone else's shit and making it my own.

Fast forward to today, I now fluctuate from 160lbs to 180lbs, depending. I love my body. I love my scars. I love my butt dimples and I especially love my Ethiopian looking, slightly droopy boobs! It has taken me 10 years to get to today and it feels amazing. It's been a beautiful journey, that all started with a simple choice. Can you believe that? Choice is such a potent thing you can really use to create anything, especially with your body.

Let me share a secret with you. Your body is magical, your butt is magical, and your breast are surely magical! You can create a million different things with them if you choose to. Money, jobs, relationship… Your body & breast desire to be included. Have you ever asked what contribution your breast be to your life today?

Yes, breast, boobies, titties, tata's… I said it! Since this is a breast book, we should dive more into the topic at hand. Breasts are defined as either of the two soft, protruding organs on the upper front of a woman's body that secrete milk after pregnancy, according to google at least.

They have been labeled differently throughout history and in different cultures with different meanings. It's quite interesting to read the judgements that surround them and opinions on which sizes were the best to have and other myths. One fun thing I have read recently was an article on how Amazon women were known to cut off one breast to become better archers! Could you imagine? I have also heard the rumor that breast were given to women by the Gods for extra armor to protect the heart in battle or fights. My favorite breast myth though, would have to be that it you have 3 nipples you are a witch! This is one is obviously true though, because I have 3 nipples. Joking, of course or am I? Either way, whatever the label or use of them are, they are pretty potent gems that can be a huge contribution to us! It really is a shame some of us don't acknowledge them more seeing as they are so lovely. *Cue playing "My Humps" by Fergie* They even have a fantastic theme song!

Personally, I was always very self-conscious about my breast. When you come from a 44DD to a 36C you tend to lose some skin tone aka have "Ethiopian boobs". I harshly judged my breasts for so many years. I was utterly embarrassed of them. I never once acknowledged them as the gift they be. I had even considered implants or a breast lift several times but it never felt right! It is a great thing that I didn't because then I wouldn't be able to share this pure magic with you!

There were two times on this path of breast appreciation that I had a strong awareness of how precious and beautiful my breasts were. The first time was during an exchange of photos between a male and I. Risky, right? (Insert scandalous laugh) He had requested that I send a picture of my breasts without my head involved to protect my identity. I asked some questions about it, and decided it would be a contribution to send the photo. Who would of thought that it would? My boobs said yes though! After I did, he responded with "No, I want a real picture! You can't just google boobs and send the first thing that pops up!" My mouth dropped, "You think I have regular normal Googlable boobs?!??" I asked. All these years I was sure they were completely screwed up and distorted! Wow! What a way to have an awesome awareness!

The following time I was in an Access Consciousness related art class and I heard them loud and clear! They wanted to be painted and used in artwork! I literally heard them screaming for it and yet I was reluctant to do it. They burned for me to, and the very thought of doing it excited me to the very core. I couldn't deny it any longer! This was an outside class so I ended up going to the bathroom with my paint and canvas. I smeared each breast with bright pink paint. The feeling of freedom that washed over me was exhilarating as I stood in the bathroom alone, pressing my breast against a canvas to make beautiful art. In those moments, I was present with my breast and my body. My being was one with my body and I took it all in a way I hadn't chosen before. I had finally acknowledged them and their beauty. As I finished up, and cleaned myself, I took my art outside to bask in the sun. It was a very empowering experience. As people commented on my painting, my breast seemed to smile. They seemed to perk up. They felt different.

What if they did change with that acknowledgement? What if it was possible to talk to and energetically lift your breast? What if it really was that easy?

Recently, with the help of the tools of Access Consciousness, I began to ask my body questions and talk to it. I told my boobs I loved them. I asked them questions, including if they could to continue to perk up! I told my breast I adored them. I touched them, I took photos and occasionally flaunted them. I gave my breast the love and attention they had been asking for. Every morning I look at my breast and body in the mirror and acknowledge every inch. My body response's accordingly. When is the last time your acknowledged or spoke to your body?

Since using these tools and having these experiences my breast and body have shifted dynamically. Everything is a different is now that I have included them in my life. I walk differently. I eat differently. I have sex differently. I do things I would have never done before! It really has been quite the journey!

Our bodies are all here for a reason. More people need to acknowledge them. Every inch of your being is here for you to adore, to speak to and to contribute to you. What magic can your breast be to you today? Have you asked? What else is possible if you did? Is now the time to include your breast in your magical life? I wonder what else you can create in this world with them? Just ask and "Breast Easy!" kids!

Brittany Rogozinski

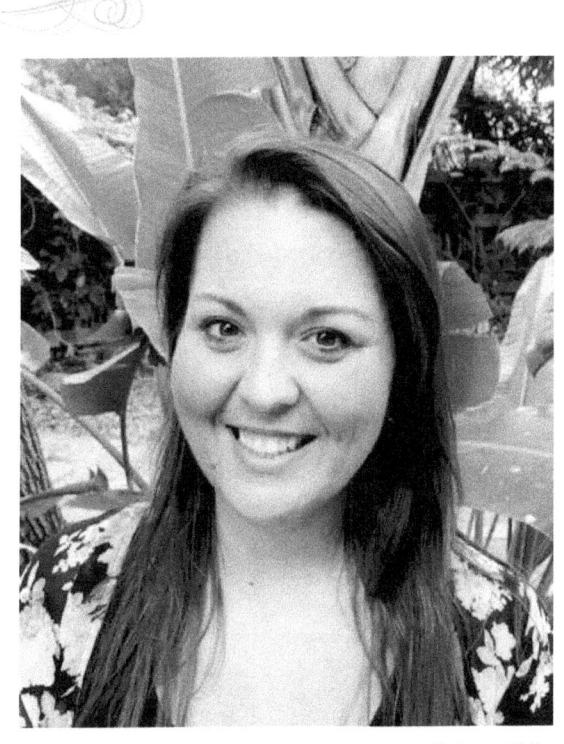

Brittany Rogozinski *has always been a creator of magnitude. From as long as she can remember things would coincidentally happen to her. From a young age she was labeled as the bad child. Growing up obese and teased, she was excluded by her family and peers. Born and raised in Bethel Park, pa, a suburb of Pittsburgh she took up medical management and used it in the weight loss field. She since has went on to become an access bars practitioner and facilitator and practices out of the Pittsburgh, PA area. She enjoys writing, poetry, graphic design and exercise in her spare time. Her target is to always live in the present.*

CHAPTER 12
BOSOM BUDDIES: BECOMING BFFS WITH YOUR BREASTS

Julie Oreson Perkins, CLC, ACC, CFMW

I'd like to introduce you to my two BFFs (Best Friends Forever): my "Girls." We've been together for several decades now – and on many adventures. Ours is a wonderful relationship, filled with ease and communion – now, that is. How did we get to this space? I'm happy to share our unique history with you, as ours is one from a completely different perspective – that of energy!

But first, I'm going to invite you to pause for a minute: Relax – breathe in fully – and exhale slowly. Do this a couple more times, please, while pondering these questions:

- Have I acknowledged my breasts as the gift that they truly are? If not, will I do so in this moment? (If YES, please acknowledge them NOW!)

- When was the last time I thanked them (and my whole body) for being with me, no matter what? Am I willing to be grateful for them in this moment? (If YES, please thank them NOW!)

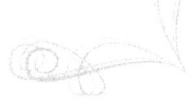

- What would it take for me to become more aware of the contribution that my breasts are to my life and living?

What did you experience just now?

I've done this exercise with many of my coaching clients who are now breast cancer survivors, who have experienced a deeper connection with their breasts – plus some (and more!) relaxation and insights into their relationship with their Girls. Even those who have lost some or all of their physical breasts to disease, damage or surgeries, have been able to experience the energy of their breasts by being completely present with them in this way.

For me, this exercise was the beginning of my current amazing relationship with my breasts…it started to open the doors to more possibilities that had been closed since my teen years.

Name Calling

As I look back, the energetic distance that got created between me and my breasts began innocently enough during my teen years. While all of my teen peers were experiencing hormones of magnitude, only half of us started growing breasts (with the exception of a few heavier boys, who developed breasts and suffered great ridicule and name calling because of that, unfortunately. I'll talk more about men and mammaries later on.) As we youthful females started "poking out and into" the world of adult women (since the appearance of breasts means you're instantly a woman, right?), we tried to make light of this "rite of passage" by calling our breasts by various names.

Some names were affectionate (sweet melons, lovely ladies, boobies)… some were given to us by the boys or men in our lives over time (hooters, titties, gazongas, headlights, knockers, tatas)… and one of my personal favorites was the name that I adopted after seeing *Carrie*, my first R-rated movie (based on the novel by Stephen King): Dirty Pillows! Carrie's mom, a domineering, highly religious person, intensely states (while the camera is focused on Carrie's chest in her prom dress), "I can see your Dirty Pillows. Everyone will." Carrie indignantly replies, "Breasts, Momma. They're called breasts. And every woman has them." That scene struck me as funny for unknown reasons, so I went through a period of calling my breasts Dirty Pillows – without realizing that there was a "shame" or "judgment" undertone in the energy that I adopted as part of that name calling.

Apparently, that "breast name calling" and the accompanying underlying energy (whether it's conscious or unconscious) continues today amongst teens. When I asked my teen daughter how she felt about her breasts, she said, "I know that boobs are supposed to be sisters, not twins – yet my bitches don't even look like friends!" It was so interesting to hear her talk about her breasts in that way. And with her statement, I was aware of how much she was comparing her breasts to each other – and to those of the rest of her peers! I was also aware that this "comparison universe" didn't stop at her breasts – the judgments continued onto the rest of her body as I noticed her wearing padded bras early on (something familiar that I remembered from my teen peers: make the boobs look bigger, so the waist appears smaller and the body shape becomes more proportionate and acceptable.) I also observed her staring into the mirror at other body parts with those same judging eyes. I wonder where she learned how to do that?

Judgment Pile Up

If I were being totally honest, I have spent DECADES judging my breasts (and body.) No wonder my daughter was doing that too! As a teen, I was the most buxom of my brood – something that I inherited from the women in my family, I was told. I remember looking at some of my grandma's party attire (she did a lot of cruises after she was widowed) and commenting, "Wow, what a busty babe she is!" I also recall wondering if I was going to be the same way? Well, I did develop breasts EARLY – and in a BIG way. (And so the foundation was laid for many layers of judgment to be piled upon…)

By the time I was in college, my upper back had become increasingly strained by the growing weight of my breasts, impacting my part-time and summer jobs as a lifeguard (swimsuits just couldn't render effective support for them, so I often had pain.) Plus, I felt fat and like my breasts were the only thing noticed about me. I decided that this needed to change, so I chose to have breast reduction surgery. During the surgery, pounds of flesh and fatty, cyst-prone tissue were removed. Somewhere I KNEW that this choice would serve me well in the long run, yet at the same time I was doubting the decision. I waffled between following my knowing that it was right for me and judging it as wrong – drastic – and sacrilegious to "mess with what God gave you." (More layers of judgement... perhaps the energy of the hospital named after a Catholic saint contributed to those layers?)

And then the astonishing (to me, anyway) aftermath of the surgery: my Girls felt perkier and rested higher on my chest – I was proud to display them – AND I felt so much lighter energetically. It was like the decrease of physical breast weight had knocked off some of the energetically-charged weight of judgment. When healed and back on campus, many people commented how great I looked, wondering if I got a haircut? Or lost a bunch of weight? (In a way I did, just not how they were thinking!) Or started working out, with great results? Even though these were seemingly positive statements, they were still energetic judgments, the implication being that something had needed improvement and had gotten better while I was away. Interesting, huh?

The Eyes Lie

The judgment pile up continued. In my early 40's, I was diagnosed with breast cancer. I was overwhelmed with parenting, running my own business as a corporate training consultant and being the manager of the house, sports teams and scout groups. I had been trying to get all of my jobs "right" including taking care of myself because "God forbid that something happened to me, the whole family would fall apart." (No judgment there, eh?) What I was most obsessed with was getting my sagging breasts and my body "back" to the "way we were" before bearing and breastfeeding children. I did this by lobbing a large amount of judgment at them daily. Each time I couldn't fit into a favorite shirt or pair of jeans – or every time I passed a mirror – I literally lasered my breasts and body with skewers of judgment, thinking and wishing that would change how they looked.

The problem was that my ideal booby and body image had been created by all the years of my eyes registering and my brain storing a multitude of pictures of what perfect breasts and bodies looked like: firm – fit – toned – and oh so healthy because of all of those gym workouts and nutritionally-sound diets. I couldn't understand why I couldn't just project that image onto my Girls and body, and get them to look that way. That's what I mean by the Eyes Lie; my eyes were simply receivers of information that just wasn't' true for me, my Girls or my body. They were soaking up all the lies from society, the media and this reality – and I was buying them like crazy. And then I made things worse by turning my eyes into transmitters of those judgmental lies, wielding them like weapons against my bosom buddies.

So in a sense, all of this judgment did actually change things. Over the course of decades, it trained my eyes, Girls and body to receive the lies and create from the energy of judgement, which resulted in massive amounts of bodily, especially boob-ily, stress. While there are many definitions of the word stress, my favorites are:

1. a constraining force or influence
2. the deformation caused in a body by such a force
3. physical, chemical, emotional (and I would add energetic) factors that cause bodily or mental tensions that may be factors in disease causation

Disease causation… in other words, the cause of not (also known as "dis") ease.

Crap. This revelation landed heavily in my world like a ton of bricks. The energy of "dying to be a perfect me with perfect boobs and a perfect body" was literally creating a life threatening dis-ease called cancer. Wow, right? Stay tuned for more about this…

Seeing What's True for Me

No matter how many years go by, I will always remember the moment that I found my breast lump. I had a normal and clear mammogram about 2 months prior, yet something COMPELLED me to do my own breast self-exam that day in the shower. Methodically palpating my right breast in circles, I felt it, nearly under my arm pit…and that's when my "eyesight" shifted. Instead of seeing my breasts through my own lie-laden eyes as sorry, sad and all washed up, I was suddenly seeing them through the eyes of doctors, healers and medicine. This allowed me to instantly see the truth – that this lump was something that needed immediate attention.

So I called a doctor that I really trusted. When his nurse answered, I explained my situation and my desire to see him immediately. She replied that there were no routine appointments available for over a month. I admit that I panicked a bit, then quickly refocused my sights on my desired outcome: an appointment with him as soon as possible. Then as if by magic, she said, "Oh wait! Somebody just passed me a note that today's staff meeting at 2 pm is cancelled…do you want to come in then?"

The magic continued as my doctor and I met – agreed to watch the lump for a month (and not panic, until we had more data) – and saw each other again in a month, when we decided to have it looked at by a surgeon. In just 30-days' time, the lump had changed shape and migrated up to the top of the skin causing mild bruising (almost like it was trying to pop itself out!) When the surgeon's scheduler said there were no appointments for yet another whole month, the magic showed up again in the form of a "just showed up in the system" cancellation for the next day.

So once again, my Girls were going under the knife – yet this time, it didn't feel like a proactive choice. It totally felt like a reaction of fear and anxiety, yet I knew it was required to get the data to support what I already knew: I had breast cancer. That was the truth and I knew it with every cell of my boobs and body. I could see that clearly.

The subsequent biopsy and lumpectomy confirmed that. The chemotherapy (that I reluctantly chose because of the side effects) and radiation (that I wholeheartedly chose, because it just made more sense to me) took care of the rest. And the best part was that because of the reduction surgery in my teens, much of the same kind of tissue that developed cancer had already been removed. So biologically and from a medical standpoint, I was in good shape. Energetically, however, I sensed that I still had some deep work to do.

Mammary Memories

If you ask any female, chances are that she will remember the time when she first realized that she had "breasts" – a tingle in the chest area, a tenderness when touched there, a show of bumps under a shirt, a curiosity about those round, reddish or brownish circles! She may also recall the accompanying emotions that came along with these developments: excitement – anxiety – uncertainty – or a feeling of "FINALLY, you've arrived!" That experience may have been influenced by her mother, sister or other female family members – her peers – her society or culture.

Ladies, whatever your experience was – good or bad – are you willing to release those memories now? "For what reason?" you may be asking… allow me to explain.

As mentioned, I was becoming increasingly aware of all that "heavy" energy and judgment projected onto or assimilated into my breasts over the years… and how utterly unkind that was to them and the rest of my body. Early teenage judgments ("They're bigger than the other girls' boobs") and the post-surgery judgment in college ("Wow, that breast reduction surgery left a lot of scars – I feel like Franken-booby now.") plus judgments as a new mom ("If I hadn't had that surgery, I would probably have more breast milk to feed my baby…") all took their toll on my Girls.

The more that I pondered those judgments, evoking memory after memory, the more my breasts "reacted." I could feel tension, anxiety and total angst in my chest area. So I chose to experiment: What would happen if I stopped this frequent rumination? And released those "mammary memories"?

Here's what I tried – and I'm inviting you to try this easy experiment with me now. Simply hold out your hands – or better yet, place them on your breasts or chest – and on the count of three, imagine ALL those "Mammary Memories" – whether they are good or bad or right or wrong – dissipating with speed and ease. And a 1… and a 2… and a 3!!! 1 – 2 – 3!!!

What did you notice? Keep experimenting. Add more 1-2-3's now. What's happening?

Even you guys can try this. Especially since I've come to realize that anything that we've held "close to our hearts" can impact the breast area and cause dis-ease. Think about it: if you were a boy teased for having breasts, you'd likely try to cover up or hide them (potentially creating a shame space in the chest area.) If you're a person who feels deeply, you're likely to pull all those emotions towards your heart space. In some countries and cultures, oaths or promises are made by placing a hand over the heart and swearing to forever do or be something (which can create solid or dense energy, if it's done out of obligation instead of choice.) And what do parents do when their child is hurting? They draw him or her close to their chests, often taking on his or her pain in order to soothe. This can happen to both females and males alike – which is why I feel it's so important for everyone to release those mammary memories. For me, when I do this (even to this day, years after my breast cancer journey), my breasts feel much less heavy and dense. This release is always a welcome relief to my Girls who I have put through so very much. (Sorry, Girls – here's an extra 1-2-3 for you and me!!!)

Tool: Interesting Point of View

Now that more of my Mammary Memories are gone – and yours are now going away too – I'm hoping that you can look at all those judgments of the past, as just an Interesting Point Of View (IPOV)! So, what exactly is IPOV?

IPOV is a personal favorite of mine from Access Consciousness®, pragmatic tools for changing your life and empowering you to know what you truly know. A Point Of View is a particular way of looking at something – and energetically, a Point Of View creates your reality. So, any opinion is a point of view – and judgments are too.

In my case, my past opinions and judgments of my breasts were based in negativity – fear – doubt – guilt – shame – regret – harsh criticism – and more…what kind of reality was I creating with those? Basically, I had created an energetically "toxic" environment for my Girls. I was projecting all of that into my world and theirs, and soon we started becoming an energetic toxicity that was literally killing us. That's what I meant earlier about creating my cancer – cute but not so bright on my part, huh? Well, once I realized that I had created it, I knew that I could un-create it by changing my Points of View.

Next time you find yourself "reacting" to something, pause – acknowledge that you are "re-acting" to someone or something (re-playing it energetically, in a sense) – and then say, "Interesting Point of View that I have this Point of View." Hint: Re-action is usually a form of judgment, like, "That idiot cut me off while driving" or "Why would he do something so stupid?" and so on. So be on the lookout for hidden judgments that surface during certain situations!

Keep saying, "Interesting Point of View that I have this Point of View" until the energetic charge (the anger or the judgment, etc.) dissipates. When you can observe that same situation without reaction, you know you're free of its energetic hold on you. Congratulations! (Want to get totally free? Continue IPOV'ing everything for 6 months and see what that creates for you and your breast friends!)

The Way Forward

Changing my Points of View plus releasing judgments and past memories has created so much more space and energy around my breasts and my body. I am happier and healthier than I've been in years and there's such a sense of ease in my daily life. Even when some of life's more difficult challenges come my way, I'm able to rise up to meet most of them by staying present and using the IPOV tool.

And it takes practice – like building muscle – so keep moving forward and stick with it. If you find yourself not making any progress, try asking a question – one that will bring up the energy of the situation so that you can look at it with "your truth" eyes and gain some awareness. Always ask generative questions, not judgmental ones. For example, "What's wrong with me? Or this situation?" is a judgment. Instead, try asking these two favorite questions of mine: "What else is possible here that I haven't yet imagined?" or "What's right about this that I'm not yet getting?"

Becoming Bosom Buddies

Here's a recap my Top 5 ways to become Best Friends Forever (BFFs) with your Breasts:

1. Be mindful of the names your call your breasts and the words you use to describe them. These names and words each have an energy of their own. Ask yourself, "Is this the energy I want to associate with these Breast Friends of mine?" (Pun intended!)

2. Quit judging yourself, your breasts, your body – immediately! Hopefully, my stories uncovered for you some of the hidden ways in which I was judging myself and my Girls – so that you can become more aware of where you may be doing the same. And now that we're all more aware of the role that judgment plays in dis-ease, let's stop judgment all together, shall we? Are you ready to take on that challenge with me? (If YES, thanks in advance!)

3. Stop viewing you through the eyes of lies. Now, please! If doing this is challenging initially, try looking at yourself or the situation through others' eyes to gain a different perspective. That difference can create enough space for you to move forward and choose differently, instead of staying stuck.

4. Release Mammary Memories: Do a bunch of 1-2-3's with your hands on your breasts or chest to release them. Still not convinced this will work? I challenge you to do it 10 times a day for 5 days to see what that creates. I dare you!

5. Use the Interesting Point of View (IPOV) tool from Access Consciousness®. Play with this tool. Flex and build this muscle. You won't regret it. But don't take my word for it. Try it for yourself. I double dare you!

Remember to have FUN while you're doing these! If what I've shared has contributed to more ease and communion with your breasts, please share your story with me at info@JulieOPerkins.com!

Julie Oreson Perkins,
CLC, ACC, CFMW

(www.JulieOPerkins.com)

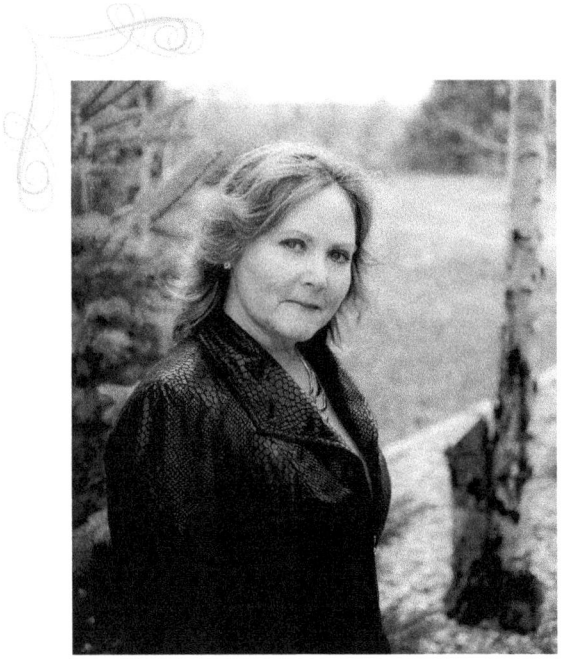

Since her first trip abroad in 1980 as an exchange student, Julie Oreson Perkins has been engaging in life-changing conversations (in several languages, including the language of energy!) with people all around the world. Today she continues her love of travel; facilitating training programs, coaching clients and speaking to groups about bringing more consciousness into the world.

Hundreds have benefitted from her "conversations of change" as a coach, teacher, motivational speaker, radio show host, international best-selling author, energy worker/healer, breast cancer sur-thriver and shamanic practitioner. These conversations result in a (re)birth of natural, intuitive abilities and zest for life on Planet Earth here and now – plus a greater connection between the Mind, Body and Soul. She's a Certified Life Coach (CLC) with an Associate Certified Coach (ACC) credential from the International Coach Federation (ICF), with specialties in Energy Leadership, Life Transitions and Academic Life Coaching for Teens. As an Access Consciousness Facilitator for Bars®, Body Processes, Energetic Facelifts and Right Body for You classes, Julie is known for her highly intuitive and dynamic energetic capacities to work with clients' bodies.

Julie is currently living in the mountains of southern California for a while, enjoying the peaceful, natural beauty there. She often takes clients outdoors to show them different perspectives, possibilities and choices without judgment, since that doesn't exist in Nature. Always the artist, she loves to create handicrafts like hand-painted silk scarves and scrapbooks of her own photographs. She's someone different: she's happy – healthy and wealthy – a purveyor of possibilities – passionate about living (and dying) consciously – AND she's an invitation to all of that AND MORE for herself, her family, her clients and her communities.

Visit www.JulieOPerkins.com or email info@JulieOPerkins.com to find out more about Julie's coaching packages – to schedule a coaching or body-based energy session – or to book her for a speaking engagement.

CHAPTER 13
THE KEY TO LOVING THE GODDESS YOU BE

Tanya Desaulniers

*W*hat if you could really, really love you? Not the mantra reciting, cliche kind, fake it till you make it kind of love you, but really undoubtedly with so much honour trust vulnerability allowance and gratitude truly love you. Every juicy morsel of you? How much fun would that be? How much ease would that be and how much more could you create in your life if you had that? And what if I told you today that I really know how we can love ourselves that much? What if there is a major key ingredient that if you committed to it, would create the true loving you and your body that you desire?

See, we chose embodiment in this lifetime. Embodiment…what the heck does that even mean? Well, we are infinite beings and therefore we don't actually require a body. We chose these gorgeous meat suits in this reality as our vehicle in this lifetime. Without our bodies, we would never feel the warmth of the sun, the wind, the cold; we would never know an orgasm, taste exquisite desserts, or feel the ocean splash upon our skin. Without these amazing smokin' hot meat suits, we would not be able to experience the loving touch of another or the exuberant rush of jumping from an airplane. They're pretty special, aren't they? They can be our best friend and number one co-creator, but so many of us are walking around, cut off at the head… ignoring the greatest ally we could ever know.

I say "No More!" Let's love us to the fullest and optimum and rock the shit out of this embodiment thing. Who's with me? See, I know that I am a mother-fucking goddess of pure Magic, and so are you. Maybe nobody ever told you that, or maybe you forgot; and I am here to remind you of the truth and make sure it sticks. We are goddesses by our very birthright, and it is time to claim, know and own that capacity now.

First, I'd like to share that I did not always love and celebrate me. I did not always love my luscious, delicious body…no way. I was born into a dysfunctional family, where loving you and your body was definitely not a part of my upbringing. Even the idea of sex was a faux pas in my home. If there was a hint of sex on the TV, my father was so immediately irate and up and left the room. I am 42 years old…so there was not a lot of sex on TV when I was a little girl..but still it triggered him. I watched this as a little child and learned that sex was dirty and not something that we should think about or talk about. No way!

I overheard my father call people names like "filthy c***sucker," which although I had no clue what that was at the time, it massively distorted the idea of oral sex for me as I got older. My parents became Born Again Christians when I was eight years old, and in the Church, are we taught to love ourselves and love our bodies? Hell No! We are taught to love God and Jesus, and put everything else before ourselves. But loving our bodies is immediately associated with inappropriate sexual behaviour. The idea of loving yourself and your body is made very clear to be Bad and Wrong, at a very young age.

I loved learning about Jesus and how He loved us, and I always felt such a love from Jesus. And then we reached and age where everything switched to the fear-pumping wrath of God, and religion no longer rang true for me. One thing that I loved, that we were taught as children, is that our body is our temple that houses our magnificent Spirit. In truth, our Spirit expands infinitely, beyond the universes. But the teachings about our body temple were so beautiful to me. I always imagined my body as a beautiful radiant temple. I would close my eyes and see lots of shining gold in my temple. My temple was always filled with jewels and with love. So, so much love. I so enjoyed imagining this temple that I naturally Be. And hey, what a cool place for a Goddess to hang out!

In Grade five, a boy from school phoned my home, to tell me that another boy had a crush on me. I was a shy little girl who blushed and hung up the phone. When I did, my father was standing immediately behind me, questioning and judging me. He asked me "What did you do to encourage this?"

Another lesson in what was bad and wrong in my father's eyes, and another way that I learned to judge the crap out of me.

I was made fun of as a young girl for being too skinny, no boobies, having acne and the braces came on in Grade 6 as well… How does it get any better than that? I knew that boys did not find me beautiful or attractive, and with the very strict rules of my home, I was not allowed to wear makeup, polish my nails, pierce my ears; or any of the things that I so wanted to be and do.

At 14 years old, I sat in front of my mirror, in my bedroom, and I cried to God, asking him why he made me so ugly. I would look at the fashion magazines and compare myself to the models. I compared myself to the popular girls at school whom the boys liked, and I just didn't measure up.

Something about me was never good enough. My body, my boobs, my bum, my face, my hair… and I concluded that I was ugly. I was not beautiful, and I wondered if I ever could be.

Well, things change, braces come off, acne clears up, boobs grow, curves fill-out, and BOOM, by the end of Grade 10, I was sought-after by the very boys who had picked on me when I was younger. I was pretty! Wow, me? I was like a kid in a candy store. The world was my oyster, and I could have my pick of pretty much any boy around. Yahoo... jackpot!

I joyously began dating and experiencing the joy of embodiment more. Well, mostly the joy of sex, but I was learning and growing. Then, three short months after celebrating my Sweet 16...I became pregnant with my first amazingly miraculous daughter; and my whole life, body and universe was forever changed and forever blessed. The day I held her in my arms, just eight days after my 17th birthday, I knew true unconditional love for the first time in my life. It was amazing and daunting at the same time, and that day I made the commitment that I would be the best Mommy I could possibly be. Today, she is 25 years old, and a drop-dead gorgeous Goddess choosing consciousness. Yay! I found her the best Daddy in the world, as I promised her I would, when she was just three years old. And, he and I are celebrating our 21st anniversary. We also have two other miraculous, Goddess daughters, who are 20 years old and 15 years old, and one magical five-year-old granddaughter. So much fun! Be careful what you wish for...lol. I always wished for girls and my whole world is girls and goddesses. We love it all... magic!

So, how else would I have created all of that magic and grown babies within my belly, if not for the gift of this phenomenally mind-blowing body and its capacities to create and heal that are still way beyond what I am currently even aware.

How could i be flying on a plane with my sexy hubby right now, to lay on a Caribbean beach, sip cocktails, play in the ocean and enjoy couple's massages together, if not for this meat suit? What a gift!

So, what if you really could love all of you, inside and out, upside or down, naked or clothed? What if? Whats the key to truly loving you? Ready...hang on to your Goddess panties because here it is. The key is never, ever, ever comparing you to anyone or anything else! It;s acknowledging now, perhaps for the very first time, that YOU are the gift this world requires. You are a piece of this magnificent puzzle. You are a integral piece, and without you, we are not a whole puzzle. See, we are all infinite oneness, and when you forget that and separate from me or others or see yourself separate from anyone or anything including the flowers or the planet or the animals; you also separate from you and the magic that you naturally be. You diminish you and your capacities to create.

So I wonder today, would you be willing to make the commitment to you, to never ever compare you to another? Would you be willing to make that demand of your right now, and therefore claim your natural right as a mother-fucking Goddess of pure magic?

Would you be willing to recognize that you are so very important, that I need you, and the Earth needs you, just as you are right now?

Now, this doesn't mean that we cannot change stuff. No way. Being grateful for you and your sweet body, does not mean that you cannot choose greater. If you are observing your bank account at a $4.00 balance, would you just sit there in gratitude, or get the fuck up and be or do whatever it takes to create some zero's behind that? Same goes for you and your body.

You get to choose and create, and choose and create, and choose again, and recreate whatever you desire. And all from a space of knowing that you can and from a space of infinite love and oneness for you and your body. Not from a place of "not good enough", or "too fat", or "too thin"; or any of that BS, that only comes from comparing you to another and judging the crap out of you. Remember, we are not doing that anymore… no way!

We are celebrating all of us, every delicious yummy scrumptious inch. Inside and out, celebrating the Goddesses we be.

Perceive this with me for a moment, if you will. What if you were the only woman alive on the planet? Just close your eyes and imagine that. What if you were the only one to commune with the Earth, animals, plants, water? What if you were the only woman here to talk to the trees and caress the grass and play with the wind? Would you have any crazy idea of fat or thin or not beautiful enough? No… you would never even know those lies or judgements. Now let's add a man (or woman, whatever floats your boat), to this image, and just imagine how he would see you. Whole and complete, amazing and magical, and his Goddess. There would be no room for anything less than that. Nobody would know comparison. What an utterly miraculous way to be and create. Yes, I am having that. Will you?

What if you choosing the magic you naturally be and loving all of you, actually heals the Earth? It does! Ask her, she will tell you. She will remind you of your potency when you forget. She never forgets. She asks only that you remember her and remember you, and reconnect with you and in turn with her as well. A very natural gifting and receiving will begin for you, the moment that you acknowledge the Goddess that you be. Stop comparing yourself to others. Choose to love you. It is mind-blowing!

A question that I love to ask is, "What energy space and consciousness can my body and I be, to be the infinite Goddess I truly be, for all eternity?"

"What energy space and consciousness can my body and I be, to be the infinite Oneness I truly be, for all eternity?"

Then I like to use this magical tool, called the Access Consciousness Clearing Statement, to just clear everything in the way of that showing up, as if by magic and at the speed of light. You can go to www.TheClearingStatement.com to learn all about it.

Over my life, I have used many different tools and forms of clearing, and nothing works like this does. It is the magic wand that eliminates all barriers and judgements, and it works! I encourage you to play with it and see what it creates for you.

So how can we change anything with our bodies with ease? Well, what if you saw her from this day on, as your best friend and ally, and actually communicated with her? What if you allowed her a voice and asked her what she likes? What touch she enjoys, what foods she loves and doesn't love, what clothes she likes to wear, what colours she would like to dye her hair? What if she loves tattoos like my sassy body does, lol, how much fun would that be?

See, bodies are super aware, often more aware than we are willing to be. If we would communicate with them and listen to their requests, we would even learn what size they love, what weight they know they would love to be, that allows them to run at full capacity and function at optimum. What if we disallowed the limitations of this reality to affect us and our yummy bodies, and started creating what we truly desire? This is an "Ask and You shall Receive Universe". All that you have to do is ask for what you desire and be in allowance of receiving it all. I love, love bodies; and I am a body communicator so bodies yap to me and often have a lot to say. Sometimes it makes me giggle. We can all listen to our bodies and create a totally new way of being together. It is all up to you. If you want a different reality and a different way of being; just choose it.

Once upon a time, about six years ago; I was sitting by the river's edge and had the clearest vision of me walking naked along the water, with long black gorgeous Goddess hair. Well, at that time, walking naked would have never happened as I had way too many judgements of me in place. I did not love me enough to gift me that ease. I also had bleached-blonde hair at the time.... Was my body showing me another possibility? Yes she was. She get's her point across loud and clear when I'm not listening, lol. See, the bleaching was destroying my hair and my body knew this. The energy of that delicious embodiment of me walking naked, was such an invitation for me to choose something greater. A couple of months later, after I had forgotten all about that vision; I missed a hair appointment and went to Wal-Mart for a box of hair dye. The one that jumped out at me was called "Very Dark Brown". It made my bleached blonde hair pure black. Yahoo! I loved it! Welcome to the dark side bitches!

Well, my very damaged hair began to grow, and today I have long gorgeous Goddess black hair, and I freaking love it. How does it get any better than that!

I do not necessarily stroll around naked much, rarely along riversides, lol, but again, it is always an energy of being and doing that we desire, and not the image in a vision. And who knows...maybe naked on the beach or by the river will be something that me and my sweet body choose sometime. What else is possible?

If losing weight is an awareness that will create more for you and your body; your body will give you a recipe as to how to be and do that and create it, starting now. Whether it's a certain kind of exercise, protein shakes, more meat, less meat, more water, less bread; whatever that is…your body is willing to be super clear and tell you exactly what she requires to create the less weight body with you.

I choose to adorn my sexy body with tattoos that my body and I choose together. We choose the design, we choose the place on my body that lights me up, and it is fun for us. What lights you up? Have you thought about it? Have you asked? Is now the time to talk to your body about it? God these meat suits are fantastic.

I am living and loving the unique Goddess that I truly be and I am refusing each day to compare any part of me to another. I am ME, all of me, and I love and celebrate me as often as I can. And I am so grateful to have a man, who chooses a love and an ease with embodiment, and looks at me like I am pure magic. How did I get so lucky?

One other important thing I wanted to remind you of, is to check in often regarding separation. Remember, when you are in judgement, you are separating from the infinite oneness that you be, and separating also from you. A Goddess knows that she is infinite oneness, and so we must acknowledge and choose that. I love to ask this question: "Am I separating right now?"

Your body will show you loud and clear, as bodies do not understand why we would ever choose the separation that we are so famous for. But, like a good and faithful servant, when we teach our bodies anything, they graciously comply. In truth, bodies love other bodies. Bodies love the interaction and love to play and love to be turned on by one-another. Bodies know that we are infinite oneness. So ask your body to make it super loud and clear when you are separating, and she will. Will you listen?

"What energy space and consciousness can my body and I be, to be the infinite Oneness we truly be, for all eternity?"

"What more could I receive right now, if i was being infinite Oneness?"

"What more could I be and receive from this person right now, if i was being infinite Oneness I truly be?"

And using the Access Consciousness Clearing statement to destroy and uncreate everything in the way of that.

Now is the time to acknowledge your magic and potency.

Now is the time to be the Goddess that you infinitely and naturally be.

Now is the time to love, honour, trust and have infinite gratitude for you.

From my heart of overflowing love and gratitude to yours; I thank you. I wonder what is infinitely, magically, miraculously, and phenomenally possible for you and your sweet body now, that was never ever possible before?

I hope to meet you in person, for hugs one day.

TANYA DESAULNIERS

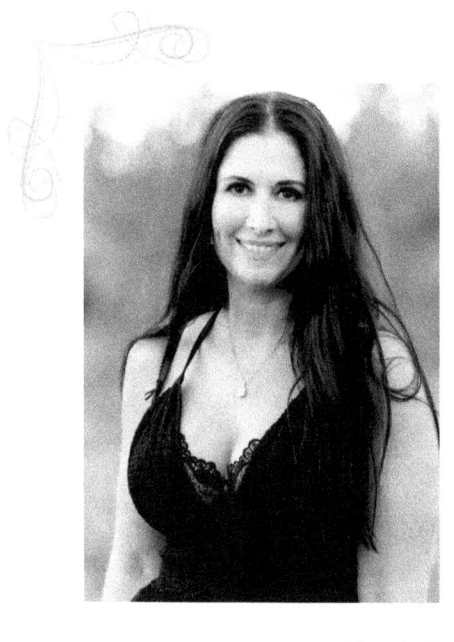

Access Consciousness Bars Practitioner and Facilitator
AC Specialty Class "Embracing Beautiful You" Facilitator
AC Specialty Class "Communion with the Earth" Facilitator
Mom and Nana extraordinaire
Sexy Wife of Consciousness, joyously co-creating magic with my amazing hubby
Infinite Being
Mother-fucking Goddess of pure Magic

CHAPTER 14
IT'S NOT EASY BEING GEE-ZY

Erica Glessing

It was this moment, I have it clearly etched in my memory. I'm riding my bike near Stanford University, where I grew up, and a boy I knew basically stopped in shock and said "Erica, what happened to you?" and it had been a full summer between seventh and eighth grade. My body changed from a lithe girl body to a curvy woman body, basically over summer!

The next memory is my dad looking in the mirror in our hallway behind me – that same summer – and he says something like "Well, what you've got, that's what all the men want," or something like that.

I basically went into a tailspin a year or two after that, gaining about 75 pounds and I never had that same innocence of girl body again. I jumped up to a DDD cup size! It was something like men looking at me, and me wanting to hide. I remember working for the ice cream store in downtown Palo Alto (Swensen's) and men would look at me with intense desire and actually call me – at that time phone numbers were still listed in the phone book – they would call and ask me out! I

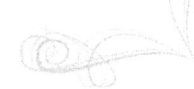

remember in college, a man somehow got my address and sent me this book, this collection of his adoration of me, and he said he couldn't help it and he was in love with me (I can't remember how he saw me, I believe it was at an event I was covering as a news reporter). So, I attracted some insanely intense attentions at that time of my life.

I learned to reject all attention. I closed off my body at that time. Something went numb. What followed was several decades of my parents trying to get me to lose weight. My mom, until her passing 15 years ago, was still suggesting I have breast reduction surgery...

On the flip side, my lovers would say "Damn you are big," when they saw my breasts. I didn't know how to accept the attention! I co-created this book "Breast Easy" to begin to ask questions about the breasts I have (G cup size now) and what might be possible that I never considered possible. I still wear big baggy clothing. Now, though, I temper the self-consciousness with a self-appreciation and self-joy because I even have a body so how lucky am I!

One of the big wake-up calls for me, working with the tools of consciousness, was that I not only turned on men but also women. Women are drawn to bodies and I didn't realize any of this until I lowered my barriers to the awareness of being in my body and allowing myself to have some ease. I started to ask different questions. So if what I was perceiving was attention from not just men, but also women, and also women whose men were looking at me – well, it's no wonder the energy around me was a firework of experience that I chose to cut off from my perception.

I was too much.

Oh! I still am! It's just now I'm harnessing my "too muchness" to change the planet bigger. There's a difference!

Your Beliefs and Your Experience

First up, I believe that my beliefs and my desires shape my experience. So, what about having in the top, say .05% of the world, in breast sizes was something I desired? What does it give me? What does it bring to me that I am joyful about? I say top .05% because given I go to the gym and given I speak in front of thousands of people, and I have three kids who play sports so I'm in arenas and rinks and I'm around a lot of people in lots of settings much of the time – I maybe see a person with breasts the same size as me every months. So, that's where I got the .05%, it's not actually scientific.

I'm also blessed with totally firm and happy and lift-y and not saggy ones. They're quite bouncy and joyful. I have a genetic line of happy breast shape. They're fun and they look good and they don't seem to be aging much as I age. They might even be getting younger. As I approach 60, I would say if you took a picture of my breasts, they act a bit more like they are about 35 or so.

So now I was asking questions, and "why" is not usually a generative question. I asked "How is this a contribution to me?" and one thing I came up with is I have a very loyal loving man in my life. I've always enjoyed loyal and loving partners and they basically don't leave. I know it's not just because of my breasts but I figure that the shape of my body has been a contribution in attracting partners who don't want to leave. I'm sure it's a combination of things but in some ways bodies do contribute and so I was looking at how lucky I am to be always able to attract lovers easily and then always able to keep lovers around easily. I can't speak to the role of the shape of my body but I figure that was a contribution I could receive when I looked at everything differently.

As I write I get this clarity around standing out in the crowd. I'm sure I stand out in the crowd whether or not my body is any particular shape. I stand out on many levels! I have exceptionally high energy, bright shining big green eyes, a joy of love and life, a big smile, big hair, a beautiful big ass, big lips, big calves, big thighs, and a zest for encouraging others to live big also. I'm also magic! And things tend to work around me. I have a knack for being able to put things together and get things together and I can learn most anything.

As I began to ask my body to contribute to the conversation instead of allowing myself to hover in the mud, slapped by parents who believed thin was the only way of being 'right' and any thickness was to be hated – as I release those concepts of self-hatred of my appearance – and ask whatever it is that I am to be a bigger contribution to the planet, everything changes. I got present to all of the people who criticized me and called me a "dog" (high school) and all of the ways that my beauty could be shrouded in clouds and shades of doubt – and as I release this, whole new horizons are possible that actually technically are quite beyond the specific curves of me.

Could You Love Yourself 1 Percent More?

It's like, could you love your body 1 percent more? Could you let your body be a contribution to your life just 1 percent more? What could you do to encourage your body to be alright, being exactly how it is?

Too Big or Too Small

When I began to formulate this book, I got present to how maybe 95 percent of women believe that their breasts aren't alright. So there was this "too small" or "too big" curse of perception that causes almost everyone to dislike the body they actually are in, right now, in this lifetime. Women who have small breasts maybe look at big ones and say "I would like some of what she's having." And women with breasts like mine might look at small ones and say "I would like some of that, some of that no need to wear a bra, some of what she's having."

So in this space of no one ever being allowed to be enough or be alright enough, there is this awareness I got of "THIS is ENOUGH," and what if what you are is exactly alright. You might have three nipples, or one bigger and one smaller breast, or maybe you have no curves at all, or maybe you have lots of curvy. What if you could look at that and ask some questions. "How is this just exactly right for right now?" and "I wonder how this body that I chose could contribute even bigger to me and my world?"

As I let down my barriers to my own brand of brilliance, I allow everyone around me to do the same. Wow. Can you sense the release of that? As you let yourself perceive your own brilliance, everything on the planet changes. Everything turns faster. It's time to let go of the places where those "slaps" from others for whatever reason can have no weight and no meaning.

Unconscious Perceptions Cut People Out of My Life

I looked at my "best" friends in high school and college, and mostly they had little to zero breasts. These were times when we were teens and we were wild and fun and danced and played basketball and we were kids. It was an unconscious thing where I hated my own shape and I was drawn to the opposite of what I was like. I gave recognition to this at one point and let down the need to friend people based on breasts (or lack there of) and I found suddenly that I wasn't noticing the breast size of any of my friends. Now, that was about 40 years ago that I chose to be friends with people who didn't have breast curves! I forgive me for that too! I wonder what unconscious things you carry around inside of you that keep you from receiving from people with different body shapes.

Look at anything that repels or attracts you with too much charge, and you can find something to release that will contribute to you having a more full life experience where people of all shapes, sizes and colors can contribute to your world.

More recently I was coaching business clients. That is something I enjoy doing a lot. I was working with clients on growing their businesses. And what showed up was an "avatar" so I teach avatar from an expansive perspective, not a narrowing perspective. It's pretty much the opposite of how avatar is taught. In so doing, I got clear on my own avatar. It's a concept where you are to tune into the audience for your work in the world. And I realized that somewhere buried deeply in my unconscious I had created my mom (who passed away) as my avatar so I could always heal her all the time.

As I released the need of my clients to look like my mom, and as I spoke to the entity of my mom and released the need to heal her still – I started suddenly meeting new clients with lots of different looks and energetic "beings" to them. Until I increased my awareness to look at what I had been attracting – I couldn't release it! Because it was stuck somewhere in between conscious and unconscious so I couldn't go beyond it.

The day after I released this "avatar" buried unconsciously, one of my clients who looked a lot like my mom cancelled our business agreement. It was so interesting. I was alright with the parting of the ways – it was light not to work with her – and this gave me space to attract new beings to play with and work with – without the unconscious draw to always heal those people who are like my mom!

New Horizons

I wonder if this book has given you any new awareness or joy that you didn't have before! I am curious if it woke up any new knowings about yourself, the beauty of you, the grace of you, the perfection of you – no matter what the size of you actually looks like!

I will tell a funny story to close that maybe you might like. One of the first group books I built had two different women authors who wrote quite similarly. That is, each submitted one chapter, and the chapters read a lot like each other's in style and substance. Both were awesome. One author was so full of herself and her chapter! She was very confident of herself and she believed strongly in her own work. In fact, she had a whole new book she was about to release and the release of the chapter book was a perfect pre-curser to her own book. Now let's go look at the other author. She was mired in self-doubt. She was sure her chapter was not a very good contribution to the book. She had been told she couldn't write for so long, and she had believed it.

From the outside (that is, from my eyes) both chapters contained major contributions and both were carefully created with a lot of insight and intelligence.

From the inside (that is, from each author's eyes) the chapters were worlds apart in quality and character.

I met with the author who was self-doubting and we looked a lot at that. I showed her how beautiful her contributing chapter was, from my eyes. She had to let go of some years of being told she couldn't write. She had to let go of self-hatred around her contributions via the written word.

What if your body was the same? Just as beautiful as every other body on the planet, just as full and rich and just as strong of a contribution? What if you could silence all those past voices of people who could not understand your beauty and your brilliance?

As you step up into your own joy, your own exuberance, your own willingness to be all that you are and all that you could be, suddenly the conversations all change!

That's the spirit of generosity I would leave you with today. The willingness to release all the judgment around you and judgment from others – and morph into the butterfly you truly be.

ERICA GLESSING

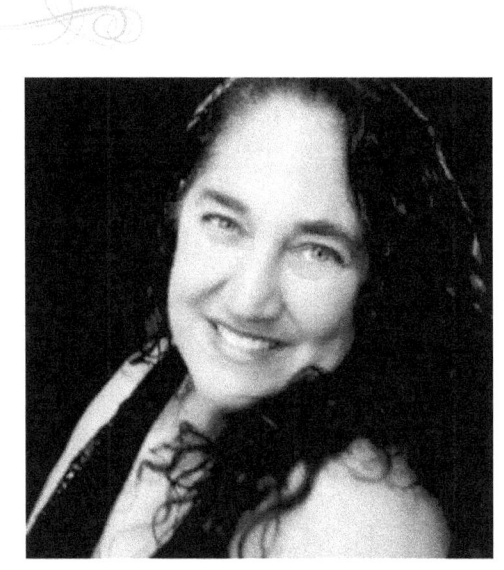

Erica believes when you tell your story, you change the world. The CEO of Happy Publishing, she is a master of happiness and creative expression. She's a #1 international best-selling author 18 times over and runs the company Happy Publishing to give light-bringers a bigger voice on the planet. In her latest book "Happiness Quotations: Generative Questions to Brighten Each Day," she brings in the power of questions to generate happiness. Find it online at www.Amazon.com and www.HappinessQuotationsTheBook.com.

You can catch up with Erica on twitter, Facebook, LinkedIn, YouTube and more @EricaGlessing and you can listen to her on her daily podcast www.TheEricaGlessingShow.com, an 8-minute daily inspirational podcast for entrepreneurs and lightworkers.

The End

www.ingramcontent.com/pod-product-compliance
Lightning Source LLC
LaVergne TN
LVHW051129080426
835510LV00018B/2310